THE WEIGHT LOSS CODE

A Practical Guide To Sustainable Weight Loss

The Weight Loss Code
A practical guide to sustainable weight loss

First Published in UK by Inspir-Her, 2020
Published in Nigeria by Worital, 2020
Edited by: Julia Bird, Tolulola Bolaji & Dayo David
Author photograph by: Camilla Harney
Cover design & layout by: Worital Global (hello@worital.com)
Copyright © Yemi Fadipe, 2020

ISBN: 978-1-8381760-1-3 (paperback)
       978-1-8381760-0-6 (eBook)

Dedication

To my Dad: Your determination to lose weight, embrace a healthy lifestyle after you were diagnosed with diabetes, and manage your health with your food is so inspiring. At first, I wondered why you made such a farce about what you ate but now thirty years on and seeing how healthy you are, I see you were right after all.

To my Mum: We started a similar project together in 2005 but I did not follow it through. I know if you are looking down from heaven, you will be immensely proud to know I finally picked it up again and this time I completed it. I love you and miss you every second of every day.

To my husband: You believe in me so much and always saw the writer in me long before I could even imagine it. I will be forever grateful to you for being such a source of encouragement.

To my kids: I believe in you and I love you to the moon and back. Never keep a skill in the bag for too long. Your gift is not for you to keep but to share with the world. Get it out there guys!

To Kenny: A friend that left us too soon. Your passing gave me the much-needed kick in the butt to start focussing on the things that matter most in life and never to waste any opportunity. R.I.P.

Testimonial

I'm intrigued by this.

When you also consider that 11% of the world population is in famine at any given time, the true figure for world obesity is being masked and is clearly higher than we are told.

So how do we address the following issues?

- Our relationship with natural and healthy food continues to diminish.
- Eating on the go or from ready prepared and convenience formats grows annually.
- Eating as a family unit is more challenged due to other lifestyle commitments and leads to poor meal choices and little meal supervision.
- Children are not educated about the benefits or enjoyment from eating healthy food. They are detached from the food chain and see healthy eating options as less fulfilling.
- Food labelling continues to be controlled by those making and marketing food and allows for poor and uninformed choices to be made by consumers.

We all know that our relationship with food has to change.

A decent, easy to follow, practical book that cuts to the chase, educates and creates a long term healthy relationship with food - written by someone who has made her own successful journey on this very path can only be a good investment.

Knowing Yemi's analytical and methodical approach I would reason that anyone with the determination to follow in her footsteps will achieve similar results to hers and I look forward to implementing some of her proven strategies and suggestions.

-Kim Palmer,
Managing Director, Staple Food Group, UK

Your free gift

As a way of saying thank you for purchasing my book, I'd like to offer you free complimentary chapters of:

The Weight Loss Code Workbook

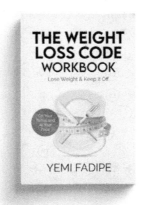

We will be covering a lot of weight loss tips and strategies in this book and I will be setting you some activities as we go. The workbook makes it easy for you to implement all the weight loss tips and strategies you will discover.

You will find everything you need to complete the activities in the book, including templates to help you assess your current weight status, to set your weight loss goal, to plan your meals and exercises, and lots more that will guide you on your way.

The paperback version of the workbook is available on Amazon and other online marketplaces.

A PDF copy of the entire workbook can be downloaded for a minimal fee from
www.weightlosscode.co.uk

Get your free complimentary workbook chapters now at
https://weightlosscodeworkbook.ck.page/

THE WEIGHT LOSS CODE BUNDLE

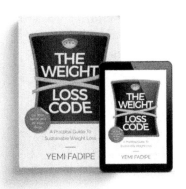

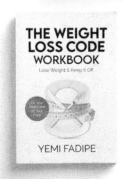 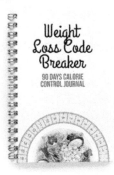

Content

Introduction

Welcome aboard an exciting weight loss adventure! If you are reading this, I know we have one thing in common – our desire to lose weight. Our reasons for wanting to lose weight may be different: to fit into a certain dress, for the perfect bikini body on our next holiday, to feel and look good, or just for the humdrum (yet important) reason of being healthy. Whatever your reason is, you have come to the right place and I can see us getting along (at least on the pages of this book). Before we get cracking, I would like to manage your expectations and let you know what you will not find in this book.

This book will not overload you with the technical jargon you hear from so-called fitness and nutritional nerds. If you are looking for technical jargon like glycaemic index, metabolic syndrome, high-density lipoprotein and any such buzzwords that make nutritionists and dieticians sound like brain surgeons or astronauts, then this is not the book for you.

Although I am a food technologist by profession, I am also your everyday girl who has tried many weight loss regimes with no luck. Finally, I came across one exciting and unrestrictive regime that simply got the job done without the help of a nutritionist, fitness trainer or dietician.

Believe me when I say I have tried many weight loss regimes. To name a few, I have tried the SlimFast 3-2-1 plan, smoothie diet, apple cider vinegar regime, ketogenic diet, and more! At some point, I was even tempted to try slimming pills. I bought them online once but never mustered enough courage to take them.

For someone of my cultural background, I should have known that I could not survive the ketogenic diet long - not eating carbohydrates for so long was like hell on earth for me. In fact, I found it very difficult to succeed in or sustain any regime based on abstinence from any particular food group.

There is nothing wrong with any of those regimes; each seemed to have worked for some other people but not for me. I have therefore concluded that there isn't a good or bad regime as such, you just need to find what works best for you and fits around your routine and lifestyle.

However, just mentioning the diets that I have tried reminds me of my many mistakes in previous attempts to lose weight. I think it is only fair that I tell you my stories around them. Not only will these stories make you laugh (I still laugh each time I remember them) but they will make you realise that you are not alone in your quest for the magic formula to weight loss.

Here goes my apple cider vinegar (ACV) story. I attended a women's retreat a few years ago and typically, the weight loss discussion surfaced during one of our chats. One of the women mentioned how apple cider vinegar had helped her lately and it did not matter what she ate, once she took her tablespoon of ACV in warm water, it increased her digestion and metabolism and she released the food quickly and easily the other way. Pardon my graphic description!

She went on to say that she had lost a ridiculous amount of weight since starting to use ACV. Then the million-dollar question popped up from another woman:

"Is there anything you can't eat when using ACV?"

Our ACV expert confidently and assuredly responded that there was nothing you cannot eat. No matter what you eat, ACV pushes it down fast.

I didn't even know what ACV stood for at the time. I quietly asked my friend who was also attending to tell me more as it appeared most of the other women knew about this magic formula. Before you know it, I became a regular customer of Holland and Barrett for ACV. I still don't know why I fell for this fad even when I did not see any difference in our ACV expert's weight at the time.

Anyway, I started using ACV religiously, following all the pack instructions as well as online recipes. I must say it benefitted me more as a home remedy for things like a cough but no weight loss occurred. I gained more weight and ended up with my teeth constantly on edge from the acidity of the product.

Then on a certain day as I scrolled through weight loss videos on YouTube, I came across a lady who claimed to have lost loads of weight in three weeks from using a mixture of turmeric, ginger and ACV. Her "before and after" images were so impressive that I convinced myself to give it a go. As I had already endured months of my teeth being on edge, I was sure I could endure another few weeks. I bought the ingredients, which included a large tub of turmeric that I still have in my spice cupboard as we speak. I followed the recipe again religiously. It tasted really disgusting but I kept drinking it anyway. Six weeks later, I was still the same tall fat girl. The only thing I noticed was I didn't catch a cold that winter as I usually did. Maybe that had something to do with the health benefits of the ingredients.

Then I travelled to Nigeria for my cousin's wedding a few months later. By this time, I weighed 93kg *(205lb/14st 9lb)* and a colleague had just told me about calorie control using an app. She was also on the weight loss roller coaster and had tried several regimes such as the Military Diet and intermittent fasting, to name a couple. I saw her lose and regain weight. So I got the feeling that some of her regimes worked but were just not sustainable. Consequently, I was willing to try calorie control. However, this trip back to Nigeria was my first since relocating to the UK nine years before. I was intending to eat all my favourite street food and traditional cuisine, from proper suya (deliciously spiced and barbecued meat on skewers), hot and fresh puff-puff (deep-fried dough balls) made on the roadsides, and snails (yes, seasoned, deep-fried giant snails in stir-fry peppers. Yum!) and more.

While in Nigeria, I hung out briefly with my Aunty Dayo, who looked fantastic at over 50 years of age. She was still as slim and beautiful as I had always known her to be. We sat next to each other at the wedding reception and I was eating everything placed in front of me. I noticed my Aunty occasionally brought out a small bottle from her bag and drank a little of the contents. This was the second time I have seen her do this. So when I visited her the next day I asked what it was about.

Aunty Dayo is one of my funniest aunts and I cannot capture your imagination well enough by translating her response into English. She told me this was her weight loss formula. She squeezed lemon or lime juice, cooked the remaining pulp for a few minutes, strained the cooked liquid and mixed it with the juice she initially expressed. This was concentrated lemon or lime juice.

"Drink this regularly and watch your body fat melt and flow away," she said, using her hand to demonstrate how the fat will flow.

"Thanks Aunty," I said, shaking my head at her unchanging humour. "I'll do it when I get back to the UK but for now I'm up for the asun (smoky, peppered goat meat chunks) your husband has just ordered for me."

As you may expect, I tried her concentrated lemon juice for a week on my return to the UK but my teeth suffered again from the acidity. Yet again, I had to give it up with no visible result.

If there is one thing I have learnt from my failed previous weight loss attempts, it is that there is no such thing as overnight weight loss. So save yourself some data space on your phone and get rid of those videos of bloggers who tell you they lost ten stones in 10 days! On the contrary, though, there is such a thing as overnight weight gain and anyone trying to lose weight knows that it is much easier and quicker to gain weight than to lose it.

Flashback to 2006: at a medical check-up a couple of weeks before getting married, I was underweight. I weighed 56kg *(123lb/8st 11lb)* at a height of 174cm and I wore size 10 (which still needed fitting sometimes). Fast-forward to 2016: in addition to getting married, having two kids and moving to another country, I had also added to my body weight. No matter how hard I tried, I continued to add more weight until I got to 93kg (205lb/14st 9lb) and started struggling to fit into a size 16.

Sustainable weight loss takes time and planned effort. Therefore, I needed to garner enough willpower to try again. This time I plunged straight into calorie control and I have not looked back. It is the best thing I have ever done for my body.

Combined with moderate exercise, I lost a whopping 23kg (50lb/3st 8lb) in six months and have successfully maintained my weight since then. If I could do it, you can too!

Prepare Your Mind

CHAPTER 1

MIND-SET FOR SUCCESSFUL WEIGHT LOSS

There are three essential ingredients for weight loss and maintaining a healthy body weight. Without these, any weight loss regime or diet plan you embark upon will end up being unsustainable and a waste of time.

Can you guess what these ingredients are?

Did I hear you say apple cider vinegar? No, not again! What about lemon juice or turmeric?

It is not any of the ingredients we have made a big fuss about in recent years: apple cider vinegar, lemon, lime, turmeric or ginger. No, not any of these.

So what are these three essential ingredients if they are not any of the above?

The ingredients are Decision, Determination and Discipline. I call these the 3Ds of weight loss.

The 3Ds of Weight Loss

1.   Decision

This is your first essential weight loss ingredient!

I am not sure about you, but I have definitely lost count of the number of people who have told me that they seriously want to do something about their weight. Unfortunately, weeks, months or even years later they are still in the exact same contemplation phase I last met them in, and still overweight! The truth is, no matter how many times I chat about weight loss, recommend solutions, share true success stories or get excited about a new diet with someone, nothing will happen until they make their own decision and begin to take decisive steps to address being overweight.

In my early days of counting calories, I was talking to my friend about this approach to weight loss. She was so excited and wanted to know more as she was already seeing the change in my weight. I gave her many useful hints and touched base with her a few days later to see if she had started. Here was the conversation that ensued between us:

Me: Have you started calorie counting? How are you finding it?

Friend: Can I really start now when I'm breastfeeding? I think I'll wait till after weaning my girl (her baby was less than six months old at the time, so what a good way to procrastinate for another six months).

Me: Uhm are you actually considering the baby or just making excuses?

Friend: uhmmmm...

Me: Would you have started last year if you'd known sooner?

Friend: Well, I was pregnant then.

Me: OK then. How about the year before that?

Friend: I was busy trying to get pregnant.

Me: Wow, you will make loads of money if you open an excuse factory. You're not ready yet.

At this time, my friend was still in the same consideration phase many people linger in endlessly with no clear action plan.

Deciding doesn't necessarily mean you have the answer or know what approach to adopt at this point but it means your mind is made up now to do something. You have committed yourself to lose weight. You are actively researching and finding useful information, putting plans in place, checking other people's success stories and have actually started thinking concretely about your next steps. It is not the planning or talking that delivers the much-needed result you want to see but the clear decision to take action.

2.   Determination

Know your WHY and tap into it. Your WHY might be as simple as fitting into a certain dress for your next party or holiday, or more health-focused like bringing down your BMI from the red zone to green zone (that was my target). Whatever your reason is, just make sure it is something that can keep you motivated. Having a goal in mind helps you to picture where you are heading. You can share your plan with a few friends or family members who are in support of your goal and can hold you accountable. Not pressure you but cheer your success and encourage you to carry on. The bitter truth of why you need a lot of determination is that not all of your friends and family will fit these criteria. In fact, to your surprise, you might find that most of these people will try to stop you because they think you are going too far, you don't need to lose weight, you are OK as you are, and so on and so forth. If you don't know or have a genuine reason (your WHY), it will be so easy to drop the ball and slip back into your old habits.

You cannot successfully go through a weight loss program just because someone you know is doing it. Having your own reason keeps you motivated. It is important though that irrespective of your reason, you set a healthy target for yourself. Check what your healthy weight range should be and make sure you are setting a target within that range and nothing lower or you will put yourself at risk of other health problems. The NHS BMI healthy weight calculator was the one I used to set my target weight *(https://www.nhs.uk/ live-well/healthy-weight/bmi-calculator/).*

Below is a picture of what my profile looked like when I decided to start losing weight, taking my weight, height, age, sex and ethnicity into consideration. I was in the red zone and decided I wanted to get back into the green zone. I set my target weight at 73kg *(160lb/11st 6lb)*, which was around mid-range of my healthy weight and gave me an allowance of 1-2kg *(2-4lb)* for special occasions like Christmas and holidays when I find it hard to stick to calorie counting. One good reason for setting a healthy target is that you know that no matter what anyone says, you are heading in the right direction. You cannot be easily discouraged every time someone says you are losing too much weight or you will become anorexic. It is your body and you know better now what is good for it.

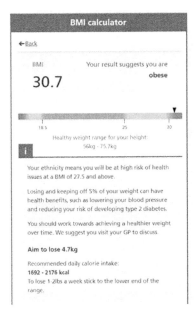

Without saying too much, I am sure you can guess my WHY. It simply was to get my weight back into the healthy range and reduce the risk of weight-related illnesses.

What is your "WHY"?
- Have a healthy BMI
- Better control of type II diabetes
- Reduce medication for cholesterol, high blood pressure and blood glucose management
- More energy and vitality
- Reduce joint pain
- Reduce back pain
- Better sleep
- Fit (back) into a smaller size clothing

3. Discipline

Discipline often gets a lot of negative publicity because it is considered as punitive, penalizing or forced abidance. My favourite of the several Cambridge dictionary definitions of discipline is:

> 'to *carefully control* the way that you *work, live,* or *behave,* especially to *achieve* a goal'

I love this definition because it summarises what sustainable weight loss is all about - carefully controlled calorie intake, adopting healthy food habits, and changing your outlook of food and behaviour around food, all in a bid to achieve a healthy weight and maintain it for the long term.

You cannot keep practicing the same old food habits with the same old inactive routine and expect a different result.

Now that you have decided to do something about your weight and are determined to follow it through, you need to stick to it, might I say "religiously". Those same old unhealthy meals will always be around you, but you now need to be disciplined enough to say "no". It is not just about removing yourself or the meal from your environment. This is not always possible, especially when you have other family members living under the same roof. You know you have made progress when despite having all those meals around, you are able to say

THE WEIGHT LOSS CODE

"no" and choose something healthier. No one says it will be easy but I know it is doable.

My temptations include the African delicacies that are always around when we meet with friends, family or even at church. Unbelievably, hardly one Sunday passes by without a celebration or another in church and there is always plenty of delicious jollof rice and fried chicken, puff-puff, and Nigerian meat pie (similar to a Cornish pasty). As if that was not enough, back home I am surrounded with my children's snacks, sweet treats and biscuits; my greatest temptation in life being shortbread. While I try to encourage healthy eating for my kids, I still cannot deny them these little treats. We don't stock up on too much of it though and they are both active kids. There is no room for PlayStations in our home so my kids are not sedentary.

My approach when I have to attend parties or functions has been to do my exercise for the day and eat my healthy calorie counted meal before leaving home. That way, I am not hungry and can select relatively healthy options from the party menu, for example, foods with few carbohydrates, more protein and plenty of vegetables, making sure the overall portion on my plate mirrors what I would eat at home. I know I will not be able to tell how many calories are in that party meal but I at least know I have kept things under control.

10

Your food temptations will be different from others depending on your personal taste, lifestyle and social life.

If you eat out regularly with friends or colleagues, you don't want to change that because you want to lose weight. That is not what we mean when we mention lifestyle changes in the context of losing weight. The bottom-line is that you need to think of those situations in advance and have a strategy for each scenario. Once when I was on a team breakfast outing with colleagues, I opted for the chef's special granola and yoghurt while there were lots of butties (indulgent breakfast sandwiches), and very alluring and tempting plates piled high with fatty foods on the table. My meal arrived last and it was so surprising to hear them say "Wow, I'd have ordered that too if I thought it'd look that good." We often fail to realise that the healthy choice can also be the tastiest choice. I also had a great time with my colleagues and that was what mattered the most.

Your lifestyle changes will be mainly around your food choices, activity level, and your perception and behaviour around food.

Friends and family will soon recognise what you are doing and stop passing comments when they see it's working for you and you don't budge each time someone tries to kindly force you to take more.

While I was in school, we learnt about exteriority and constraint in psychology class. Exteriority is how you act and behave when you are around people and know they are watching. Constraint means those things you do while you are by yourself and know that no one is watching.

Discipline when losing weight is not so much about how you behave around food in the occasional social gatherings and parties. More importantly, it is what you do when you are on your own. You cannot keep going back to sneak unhealthy snacks from the cupboard, convincing yourself you will only do it once. You need discipline far more at home than anywhere else. It is a good idea to limit the amount of unhealthy meals, snacks, food and drinks that you stock, and better still to replace them with healthy alternatives. However, it is far better to overcome that addiction to unhealthy food and be able to show restraint even when they are all around you. It starts with baby steps and you can take it one day at a time. In a few weeks, you will find this begins to become second nature.

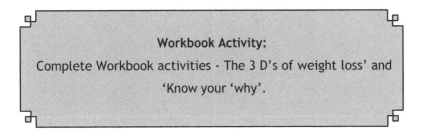

Workbook Activity:
Complete Workbook activities - The 3 D's of weight loss' and 'Know your 'why'.

SECTION 2

Everything You Need to Know

CHAPTER 2

YOU ARE ALLOWED TO EAT

Yes you are! You might find it strange to see a heading like this in a book about weight loss and healthy eating. However, it is true that you are allowed to eat any food. There is no such thing as bad food, only bad quantities (portion sizes).

Permit me to take you back to elementary science or biology when we learnt the importance of nutrients. Can you still remember it? I would understand if you have forgotten but now let us jog our memory with some basic nutrition.

1. *Carbohydrate provides energy for the body. It can be found in all starchy foods, such as bread, rice, potatoes, pasta and breakfast cereals; but also in simpler forms as the sugars present in fruits, vegetables and milk.*

2. *Dietary fibre is important for our health and for reducing the risk of some diseases (e.g. heart disease, type 2 diabetes and colon cancer). It also helps our digestive health and reduces the risk of constipation. It can be found in high-fibre breakfast cereals, whole grain bread, whole-wheat pasta, beans, pulses, fruit and vegetables.*

3. *Protein provides amino acids, some of which we cannot make ourselves and so need to get from our diet. It is needed for normal growth and maintenance of health, and provides energy. It is found in meat, fish, eggs, dairy foods, cereal products, soya products, nuts and pulses.*

4. *Fat provides essential fatty acids (that we cannot make ourselves but need in small amounts) as well as energy. It is required for a range of bodily processes and to maintain the normal structure of cells in the body. It also carries essential fat-soluble vitamins and is important for their absorption. Sources include fats and oils, meat and meat products, dairy foods, oily fish, nuts, seeds and avocado.*

5. *Vitamin B1 helps to release energy from food. It also helps our nervous system and heart function normally. Sources include bread, fortified breakfast cereals, nuts and seeds, meat (especially pork), beans and peas.*

6. *Vitamin C helps to protect cells from damage. Helps with the formation of collagen, which is important for normal bones, gums, teeth and skin. It also helps the immune system work as it should and the nervous system to function normally. It is found in fruits (especially citrus fruits, blackcurrants, strawberries, papaya and kiwi), green vegetables, peppers and tomatoes.*

7. *Vitamin D helps the body to absorb calcium and helps to keep bones strong. It also helps muscles and the immune system to function normally. It is found in oily fish, eggs, fortified breakfast cereals and fat spreads. In summer, the majority of people will get most of their vitamin D through the action of sunlight on the skin.*

8. *Vitamin E helps to protect the cells in our bodies against damage. It is found in vegetable and seed oils (e.g. olive, rapeseed, sunflower, peanut oils) nuts and seeds (e.g. sunflower seeds and almonds), avocados and olives.*
(Source: the British Nutrition Foundation. ExploringNutrients. https://www.nutrition.org.uk/healthyliving/basics/ exploring-nutrients.html?start=2, accessed June 22, 2020)

In the extract above, I just selected the macronutrients and a few micronutrients to show you the good that each one does for the body. Macronutrients are those nutrients the body needs in large quantities because they provide energy and are the building blocks for the body's growth and maintenance. That includes mainly protein, carbohydrate and fat. Micronutrients on the other hand are those needed by the body in small amounts but are highly essential for the body to work properly. Vitamins and minerals belong to this category.

If you want to learn more about this, you may want to look up the British Nutrition Foundation website.

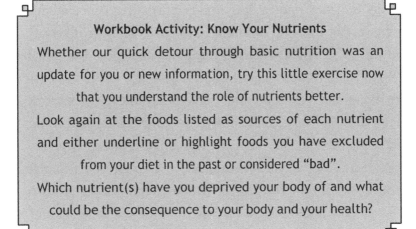

Workbook Activity: Know Your Nutrients

Whether our quick detour through basic nutrition was an update for you or new information, try this little exercise now that you understand the role of nutrients better.

Look again at the foods listed as sources of each nutrient and either underline or highlight foods you have excluded from your diet in the past or considered "bad".

Which nutrient(s) have you deprived your body of and what could be the consequence to your body and your health?

How many can you see? I can straight away see bread, pasta, breakfast cereals, meat and eggs. Yes, eggs! I grew up with the impression that eating eggs was bad for your heart. Even fat is essential for health.

The take home message from this quick memory refresher is that there is no bad food as such (as controversial as that may sound). The nutrients we need to keep healthy come from wide and varied food groups and so our diet needs to be diverse and include many of these different foods in the right proportion. Did you see the key phrase there? THE RIGHT PROPORTION.

There are foods that we need to eat more of and those we need to eat less of. Every nutrient has a part to play in keeping us healthy and our bodies functioning normally. This explains why I am not inclined to follow a diet plan that excludes any nutrient or outrightly restricts any particular food. Diets that exclude certain food groups or nutrients are likely to cause nutritional deficiencies, which have undesirable effects such as the loss of energy, an inability to concentrate and other health problems. This makes them unsustainable over the long term. Also, if you are not allowed to eat a particular favourite food, your body will crave the excluded food so much that you eventually bow to its cravings and you will consume it excessively. In essence, if you are going to lose weight and maintain a healthy weight for the long term, what you need is a BALANCED DIET – food in the right mix and proportion for you.

I am sure your next question is; what then is the right balance for me? You need to trust the experts here and what the experts say is that an average woman needs about 2000kcal and a man 2500kcal daily from all foods and drinks to maintain their weight. This should comprise:

- At least 5 portions of fruit and vegetables
- 3-4 portions of carbohydrates
- 2-3 portions of protein foods
- 2-3 portions of dairy or alternatives
- Very small amount of oils and spreads

The simple and easy guide below was put together by Public Health England to help put this food mix into perspective visually. It is called the Eatwell Guide.

Public Health England, British Nutrition Foundation and the World Health Organization all agree on these recommendations. I trust them as well because as a food technologist, I know that they are based on extensive research and data. Not only that, but I have lost weight by correctly applying this guidance and I am going to show you just how to do the same.

So come with me: let's do this!

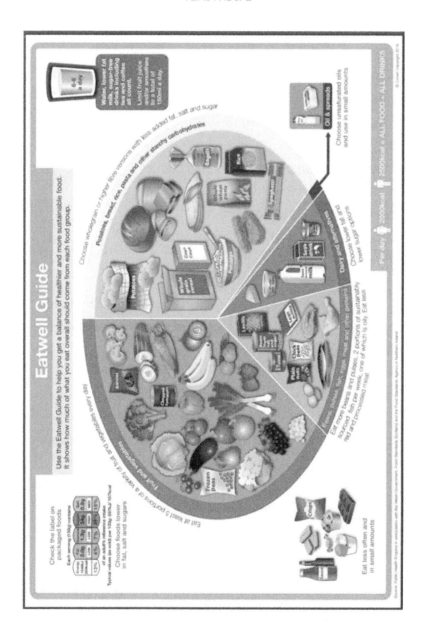

THE WEIGHT LOSS CODE

CHAPTER 3

CALORIE CONTROL 101

Before you start trying to control calories, I think it is best that you understand what it is that you are actually controlling. Let us start with the basics.

People are always throwing around the word calories – but what is a **CALORIE?**

A calorie itself is simply a unit of measurement for energy. In everyday science, it is the amount of heat needed to raise the temperature of 1 gram (0.04oz) of water by 1°C (34oF). However, when we talk about calories in relation to food, it is referring to kilocalories, which you will often see abbreviated as kcal. A kilocalorie is 1000 calories. Just like 1000 metres make 1 kilometre in distance, 1000 grams make 1 kilogram in weight, 1000 calories also make 1 kilocalorie in energy. In essence, 1kcal is the amount of energy needed to raise the temperature of 1 kilogram of water by 1°C (34oF). Don't ask me why we call them calories rather than kilocalories. I also can't stop wondering how many microseconds longer it takes to call them what they are!

With the true meaning of calories in mind then, calories in food is a measure of the amount of energy we get from the food and drinks we consume. When we consume more calories than we use, we gain weight because the excess energy is stored as fat in the body.

There is nothing wrong with fat in the body; in fact, it's an important nutrient required for many bodily functions, as we already touched on earlier. However, weight gain occurs when the fat you store exceeds what your body needs and can burn. To maintain a healthy body weight, you should only consume enough energy for your body's daily functions. Weight gain is therefore a result of sustained and continuous consumption of calories more than the recommended daily calorie intake. That is the simple science behind weight gain.

The recommended daily intake can vary for individuals depending on their activity level, age, sex and size. This is where the general advice of 2000kcal/2500kcal recommended daily calorie intake for women and men respectively come in. I will show you how to find your right daily allowance when we set your daily calorie intake target later on in the book.

Therefore, if overweight is a result of excess calories stored up as fat, then in order to lose weight, you need to reverse the equation by:

Creating a calorie deficit (consuming less than your recommended daily calories but still within a healthy range) for a sustained period
and
Burning up excess stored fat (through regular exercise)

Once you reach your target weight then you maintain it by consistently:

Keeping your daily consumption within your recommended daily calories intake
and
Daily or regularly burning up any excess calories

Can you already start to see where exercise creeps into the equation? We will tackle that too later on.

People tend to make a big deal out of what constitutes a good or bad calorie. While some foods can be healthier than others (we all know broccoli is probably better for us than chocolate), there is no such thing as a good calorie or a bad calorie. It doesn't matter whether you are feeding on green smoothies, salads or chocolate. As long as you consume more than the calories you need, you will gain weight.

In fact, I gained more weight in the years I had green smoothies as my daily breakfast than any time before or after that. The fact is, a calorie is just a calorie, whether it is from broccoli or from chocolate. It is the same as a centimetre is just a centimetre whether drawn on paper or on the floor. To implement calorie control, you need to understand how many calories you are likely to get from different foods and use that information to correctly balance your meals.

The beauty of calorie control is it does not matter what you eat. As long as you consistently do not exceed that daily calorie budget for a sustained period, you will lose weight. You will quickly find out though, that if you want to be full and not feel constantly hungry, you will need to be smart about what you eat throughout the day to make up and stay within that target calorie budget.

You need to be aware of the fat, carbohydrate and protein in foods because each one provides different levels of calories. Water is about the only thing we can consume as much as we like without worrying about calories. Pure, natural water thankfully has zero calories and is naturally present at different levels in nearly every food we eat. It is like the bottomless drink on an 'all you can eat' buffet menu. The other macronutrients will contribute to your total energy intake:

- 1 gram *(0.04oz)* of carbohydrate provides 4kcal
- 1 gram *(0.04oz)* of protein provides 4kcal
- 1 gram *(0.04oz)* of fat provides 9kcal

You can see right away why there is a lot of talk about reducing your fat intake if you want to lose or maintain a healthy weight. Fat contains more than twice as many calories per gram as carbohydrate or protein!

Based on the calories per gram shown above, if your daily calorie target was 2000kcal and one of your meals weighed 300g (11oz) equally split between fat, carbohydrate and protein, you are straight away consuming 1700kcal in a single meal. It is almost certain that you will then exceed your daily target. Just by snacking on a chocolate bar or even a small serving of almond nuts, which is supposed to be a healthy snack, you will exceed your daily calorie target.

If, on the other hand, you decide to split the same 300g (11oz) meal into three equal portions as your three-square meals for the day, you would have kept within your calorie allowance. If you repeat that consistently for a sustained period, you will start to notice a drop in your weight even within the first week. The problem here though is 100g (3.5oz) food is so small that you would be constantly hungry and probably feel like you are starving.

You therefore need to know which foods have lots of calories per gram (high calorie density), which ones have few (low calorie density), and which ones provide very little or no calories at all (very low calorie density) so you can cook well balanced meals and consume the right portion sizes.

The simple way of working this out is to check the energy per 100g on the label and divide it by 100. That gives you calorie per gram. Here is what this might look like on your food label.

Nutrition Information	
Typical values	**Per 100g**
Energy	2105kj
Energy	505kcal
Fat	25g
of which saturates	16g
Carbohydrate	62g
of which sugars	38g
Protein	5g
Salt	1g

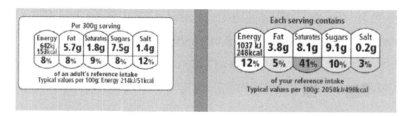

Per 300g serving

Energy 642kj 153kcal	Fat 5.7g	Saturates 1.8g	Sugars 7.5g	Salt 1.4g
8%	8%	9%	8%	12%

of an adult's reference intake
Typical values per 100g: Energy 214kJ/51kcal

Each serving contains

Energy 1037 kJ 248kcal	Fat 3.8g	Saturates 8.1g	Sugars 9.1g	Salt 0.2g
12%	5%	41%	10%	3%

of your reference intake
Typical values per 100g: 2058kJ/498kcal

For example, I have just looked up Hovis Soft White bread and it has 233kcal per 100g so the calorie density is 2.3. You can also do it using the serving size if you know the weight of a serving size. Using my Hovis soft white bread example again, each slice is 50g and provides 117kcal and the calorie density still works out as 2.3 (117kcal divided by 50g) The same approach applies if your label is expressed in ounces or other units of measurement.

Below is a list of 80 randomly selected foods categorised by their calorie density. I have done this to help you to get a good grip of where different types of food belong.

High Calorie Density (>4kcal/g) (>100kcal/oz)	Medium Calorie Density (1.5 - 4kcal/g) (37.5 - 100kcal/oz)	Low Calorie Density (0.6kcal -1.5kcal/g) (15 - 37.5 kcal/oz)	Very Low Calorie Density (<0.6kcal/g) (<15kcal/oz)
Chocolate	Chocolate cake	Wild rice	Raw carrots
Suet	Dried figs	Smoked cod	Melon fruit
Pastry	Rice-based	Roasted par-	Damsons
Pecan nuts	breakfast cereals	tridge	Papaya
Beef dripping	Pork meat	Lean beef	Gherkins
Sweet biscuits	Meat-topped	Chicken meat	Cherry tomatoes
Sunflower seeds	pizza	King prawns	Passionfruit
Butter	Oven-baked	Grilled hoki Fish	Kumquats
Peanut butter	potato chips	Mullet Fish	Brussels sprouts
Chocolate-coated	Lamb meat	Whole boiled	Lemon juice
cereal bar	Roast nut and	eggs	Apples
Cheddar cheese	seeds	Homemade	Tomato juice
Cakes	Wholegrain	guacamole	Butternut squash
Pistachio nuts	brown rice	Coley fish	Low alcohol
Hazelnuts	Grilled salmon	Homemade	cider
Roast duck	Single cream	red lentil curry	Fat-free yoghurt
Cocoa butter	Bread-	(Masoor dahl)	Guava
Sunflower oil	crumb-coated	Boiled egg	Fresh mint
Melon seeds	scampi	noodles	Artichoke
Nougat	Boiled egg yolk	Haddock fillets	Periwinkles
Olive oil	Crème fraiche	Red snapper	Broccoli
	Grilled kippers	Ricotta cheese	
	Swiss-style	Fruit mousse	
	muesli	Low fat yoghurt	
	Beef brisket	Steamed yam	
	Pea bhaji	Chickpeas	
	Scones		
	Wild salmon		

To eliminate any unconscious bias, I intentionally used a randomiser to select the foods in the table from an industry-recognised food composition database. I don't want to give you a list made up only of my familiar foods or those popular in the part of the world I live in. I wanted you to see that you can create balanced, healthy meals with foods from any culture or part of the world.

Take a closer look at the table again. Can you see any pattern? Did you notice that the very low calorie density foods are mainly fruits and vegetables; low calorie density foods are mostly white meat, fish, lean meat, pulses; medium calorie foods are mostly red meat, carbohydrates, fatty fish; and high calorie density mostly fats, oils, nuts, sweets and more carbohydrates?

Low calorie density foods are naturally more filling because they provide very few calories per gram, which means you are able to eat enough to fill you for fewer calories than eating a meal based on high calorie density foods. Take the example of one of the breakfast smoothies I used to make before I understood calorie density. Let's see how the calories compare with the like-for-like weight of one of my new favourite breakfasts: fruit bowls.

Breakfast smoothie		Breakfast fruit bowl	
1 small avocado (136g/4.8oz)	233kcal	Diced fresh pineapple (100g/3.5oz)	45kcal
1 medium banana (129g/4.6oz)	105kcal	Red seedless grapes (111g/3.9oz)	75kcal
Almond butter (20g/0.7oz)	129kcal	Diced fresh mango (100g/3.5oz)	48kcal
3 teaspoons cocoa powder (6g/0.2oz)	19kcal	Honeydew melon (100g/3.5oz)	48kcal
1 cup unsweetened almond milk (250g/8.8oz)	30kcal	Papaya (130g/4.6oz)	57kcal
Total meal weight 541g (19oz)	516kcal	Total meal weight 541g (19oz)	273kcal

Can you see how using lower calorie density ingredients brings the total calories down significantly for the same meal weight? Your meals don't have to be made up solely of low-calorie density foods. As you can already see from the calorie density table, high calorie density foods are not bad or forbidden foods. All you need do is start rebalancing your meals by increasing the amount of low calorie dense foods, using their volume advantage to keep you full and combining that with a reduced proportion of high calorie density foods to create healthy, exciting, delicious and filling meals with allowance for a few of your favourite treats to satisfy your cravings.

I am sure by now you can start to see the reasoning behind the Eatwell Guide platter we saw earlier and why the different food/nutrient sources are combined in different daily portions.

In summary, sustainable weight management is not achieved by food or nutrient deprivation. Portion control is essential, and it needs to be combined with a healthy balanced diet.

I hope I have not overloaded you with information or scared you off with scientific data! I am not expecting you to get out the calculator in the store and calculate everything before you are able to pick an item on the shelf while shopping. That certainly is not the point. I just need you to be equipped to make your own food choices and not be misled by the many fads out there. You can now begin to identify the changes you need to make to your food choices and your shopping list going forward if you are going to achieve your goal.

Workbook Activity: What's on My Plate?

Set a day aside to confirm your current breakfast, lunch and dinner portion sizes.

Before each meal:

- Make a list of the food/ingredients in the meal. Take photos of the front and back of pack label. You will need them for another activity later.
- Weigh and write down the weight of the empty plate.
- Dish up your meal as you normally do.
- Weigh and write down the weight of the dish of food.
- Subtract the weight of the empty plate from the weight of the plate of food. The difference is the weight of each meal.

Write down the weight of your breakfast, lunch and dinner for that day.

Create your own calorie density table and start putting the food/ingredients in your list into their calorie density category in the table. Use the calorie information on the label. Feel free to repeat for other food/ingredients you use regularly.

CHAPTER 4

SMART SWAPS

Why do you need "smart swaps" when I said you could eat anything you like?

Indeed, you can eat whatever you like, however depending on how soon you want to reach your target weight, you may need to swap some high calorie foods for their lower calorie equivalents. Switching to lower calorie food stretches your daily calorie budget as it allows you to get more food for less calories.

The world of weight loss is one of the few places where LESS IS MORE! Your aim when making swaps is to get more food for fewer calories, so you feel full and reduce or possibly eliminate the cravings often associated with weight loss regimes.

You crave less because in principle, you are still eating the foods you like; only this time it is their low calorie equivalent.

For instance, maybe like me you drink milky tea and coffee. Say you currently use whole milk and go through 200ml (7 fl oz) daily. That is 132kcal. Switching to any of these lower calorie equivalents or replacements will work out as follows:

- **Semi-skimmed milk, 200ml *(7 fl oz)* at 100kcal** (saving 32kcal)
- **Skimmed milk, 200ml *(7 fl oz)* at 74kcals** (saving you 58kcal for the same amount of milk)
- **Unsweetened almond milk, 200ml *(7 fl oz)* at 29kcals** (saving you a whopping 103 calories for the same amount of "milk")

This swap does not only mean you have saved some calories. It also means if you need more milk for other reasons, you would have used: nearly 1½ times the amount of semi-skimmed milk, nearly twice the amount of skimmed milk, or nearly five times the amount of unsweetened almond milk before you consume the same number of calories as you would in whole milk.

This will play out similarly in a full meal.

If you have oat porridge for breakfast daily and use 200ml *(7 fl oz)* of whole milk, switching to any of the same lower calorie equivalents will automatically take 32 –103kcal off your breakfast without you reducing your portion size. You will still be as full as you always were. If that switch was to unsweetened almond milk, over one month (with nothing else changing), you could have lost a whole pound, using the conversion of 3,500kcal per pound of body fat.

Now that is only one food swap. Imagine the impact if you took the same approach on multiple other ingredients or foods you consume regularly.

When I was losing weight, I was often asked if I always felt hungry. There was always disbelief or surprise in people's faces when I replied with an emphatic "No". At the beginning, when I was trying to stick to my daily calorie target while still consuming high calorie foods and ingredients, I had less to eat because the calories added up so quickly and I was always very hungry. I would curl up in a corner of the sofa quietly after dinner not because I was tired but because I was still hungry (yes, I did! LOL!). Then I began exploring swaps and came up with a whole lot of options that made my weight loss journey a smooth and easy sail. I also ended up learning new recipes that I loved and have become part of our family meals.

By the way, the unsweetened almond milk illustration was one of my swaps and I now mostly use it in place of milk unless it is absolutely impossible to do so. In such cases, I would go for skimmed or semi skimmed milk.

I made many other swaps, some of which I would love to share with you. I call them my Smart Swaps. This is not an exhaustive list but I hope it serves as a guide or pointer to your swapping opportunities and hopefully you find smart alternatives for your other favourite high calorie foods and ingredients.

Food	Kcal per 100g (3.50z)	My Smart Swap	Kcal per 100 g (3.50z)	Calorie savings
Butter	744	Sunflower spread light	289	45.5kcal saving per 10g (1/3 oz) serving of butter.
Mackerel fish (raw)	233	Hake fish, red bream (raw)	96	137kcal saving per 100g (3.5 oz) serving. May vary with cooking method but on a like-for-like basis you would save over 50% of the calories by swapping. Red bream is also very delicious.
Brown sugar	380	Stevia	2	98 - 100% savings here, and that is if anyone would even use 100g (3.5 oz) of stevia!
White sugar	394	Honey	288	10-19kcal per serving. This may surprise people who consume loads of honey. Honey is not a low-calorie option.
Full fat natural yoghurt	81	Fat-free natural yoghurt	48	33kcal saving per 100g (3.5 oz) serving.
Full fat Greek yoghurt	120	Fat-free Greek yoghurt	54	66kcal saving per 100g (3.5 oz) serving. This swap was a big win for me as I love Greek yoghurt so much and have it for breakfast at least 3 times a week.

Food	Kcal per 100g (3.50z)	My Smart Swap	Kcal per 100 g (3.50z)	Calorie savings
Palm oil (also contains 50g (1.8oz) saturated fat per 100g(3.5 oz)	899	Extra virgin olive oil (also contains 14g saturated fat per 100g)	884	36% reduction in saturated fat intake. *This was a good swap for my cholesterol level. This is not only about cutting down calories but also saturated fat. Oils are all highly caloric because they are naturally 100% fat so the key is to swap to a healthier oil and reduce the quantity you use in your meals.* **SWAP AND CUT!**
Vegetable oil (e.g. sunflower oil)	899	Fry light cooking spray	488	130kcal savings per serving. *Cooking sprays are brilliant. It is only 1kcal per spray and 5 spray servings is equivalent to 1 tablespoon of vegetable oil, which contains roughly 135kcal. This swap was a revelation for me in that it made me realise how much of the oil I used in cooking wasn't really needed.*
Long grain white rice	131	Basmati white rice	117	14kcal savings per 125g (4.4oz) serving. *This may seem small but this is another that is not only about saving calories. Considering*

Food	Kcal per 100g (3.50z)	My Smart Swap	Kcal per 100 g (3.50z)	Calorie savings
				rice is one of our most versatile staples, you will not only need to swap but also to reduce your portion size. If you are like me and my husband, who we nicknamed "Rice man," you probably already eat far more than 125g (4.4oz) in one meal portion. The key to keeping rice in your recipes is to **SWAP AND CUT.**
		Bulgur wheat	83	34 - 48kcal savings per 125g (4.4oz) serving. *I didn't do a complete swap from rice to bulgur but started trying out other similar grains, e.g. freekah, quinoa, couscous, pearl barley to make my meals more varied and exciting.*
Regular cola	42	Diet cola	0.4	104kcal saving per 250ml (8.5 fl oz) serving. *That's a lot for those of us who drink fizzy drinks. Some hard-core fizzy drinkers can spot the difference even if blindfolded but I have done this swap now for over 5 years and I am so used to the diet version I don't even consider the regular.*

41

Food	Kcal per 100g (3.50z)	My Smart Swap	Kcal per 100 g (3.50z)	Calorie savings
		Infused water	0 to 5	*Swap to homemade infused water is even better if you are avoiding fizzy drinks. I have done a fizzy drink **SWAP AND CUT**, so I either take the occasional diet fizzy drink, but more regularly lemon infused water that I carry with me and drink all day, even at work.*
Potato (boiled)	74	Sweet potato (boiled)	58	16kcal saving for every 100g *(3.5oz).*
White bread	93 (per slice)	Wholemeal bread	64 (per slice)	29kcal saving per slice. *This is not a real saving if you compare nutrients per 100g (3.5 oz). The savings are due to the slices being smaller. You can achieve the same savings with portion reduction on white bread, but I love keeping things simple.*
All-butter shortbread fingers	518 93 per finger	TUC or Ritz crackers	523 26 per biscuit	83 calories saving per biscuit. *This for me was unbelievable. I never ever thought cream crackers could have more*

Food	Kcal per 100g (3.50z)	My Smart Swap	Kcal per 100 g (3.50z)	Calorie savings
				*calories than my beloved shortbread fingers. Sadly, because each shortbread finger is about 19g(2/3 oz) compared to 5g (1/5 oz) for my TUC cracker and I traditionally had at least 4 fingers with tea every night, the swap to 4 crackers made sense. It saves me over 300 calories every night I sit down after the kids' bedtime to indulge in my tea and biscuit. **SWAP AND CUT***
				I hope someone from Walkers shortbread is reading this and will pleeeaaase develop a thinner shortbread slice. I'd be swapping straight back!

My most rewarding swap was replacing my deep fryer with an air fryer. Oh my goodness! This meant I did not only swap foods but also did a smart swap on cooking method, largely replacing oil frying with air when frying or grilling, except the very rare occasions where this was impossible. I am probably only left with one or two snacks and sides that I still fry in oil and they are not regular meals. I never knew some foods tasted so good until I started air frying.

> **Swap:** an outright change to a lower calorie alternative.
>
> **Cut:** is where I keep the same food but reduce my level of consumption.
>
> **Swap & Cut:** is where I swap to a more nutritious alternative but still reduce my level of consumption because the calorie content on a like-for-like weight is still comparable.

While some swaps may look like they deliver little savings on calories, they do add up quickly over time and make a lot of difference to your daily meal planning. As I concluded writing this section, I needed coffee and remembered I had a can of iced cappuccino coffee in my cupboard. I had brought this home to try and it was delicious and refreshing, but that 250ml (8.5 fl oz) can contained 153kcal, which is equivalent to about 70 cups of my regular coffee! Checking the back of the pack, I found the product contained mainly semi-skimmed milk, coffee, sugar and maltodextrin, whereas my regular cup of equally refreshing and delicious coffee would contain coffee, unsweetened almond milk and stevia. The semi-skimmed milk, sugar and maltodextrin really increased the iced coffee's calorie content, yet I enjoy my much lower calorie Smart Swap just as much.

What I am hoping to drive home in this section is that maintaining a healthy diet or controlling your calorie intake does not have to be about complete abstinence or elimination of any food from your meals, but making smart food choices, swaps and getting the portion size right.

Calorie Checkers

I will soon be asking you to find your own smart swaps but not until I have shown you where to find the information you need to make those decisions. There are many online nutrient databases with reliable, verified nutritional information on food items and ingredients. You may not find them all on one database and may need to be familiar with more than one but ultimately you will find one that contains the most information about your regular foods.

Here are some resources but it is not an exhaustive list. You can always find more and build this list further for yourself. My only request is that you ensure it is data based on verified information and not just some random blog.

- **NHS Calorie Checker**: https://www.nhs.uk/live-well/healthy-weight/calorie-checker/

- **McCance & Widdowson Foods Dataset**: https://www.gov.uk/government/publications/composition-of-foods-integrated-dataset-cofid (this a regularly updated government database that the food industry uses)

- **Food calorie counter**: https://caloriecontrol.org/healthy-weight-tool-kit/food-calorie-calculator/

- **Supermarket websites**: Product pages on supermarket websites are also a great place to check calorie information. If selling online, supermarkets are legally obliged to provide mandatory product information (which includes nutritional information)

Workbook Activity: Smart Swap Challenge

Create your own Smart Swaps for the high calorie density foods in the list you created in the previous activity. Use the calorie checker to find lower calorie alternatives. Decide what you may want to swap with and mark as Swap, Swap and Cut, or just Cut as the case may be.

THE WEIGHT LOSS CODE

CHAPTER 5

WHERE DOES IT COME IN?

I don't know about you but "exercise" was one of my least favourite words ever. It would possibly have been in my top 20 worst words in the past, but now I don't mind it so much. Having said that it's still not on the top 20 favourite words and may never be. Exercise is where the third of our 3D ingredients come in handy – DISCIPLINE.

If you asked me to choose between losing weight by either portion reduction or exercising, I would choose portion reduction every time. Unfortunately, while weight loss can happen purely with calorie control, it happens quicker and is more sustainable when combined with regular exercise. I would not go into the science behind exercise since I am not an expert in that field. Nevertheless, we have been told that exercise helps us lose more weight because it increases our metabolism and helps our body burn fat quicker.

I believe both because I have experienced them first hand on my weight loss journey. When I first started exercising, I found myself always needing the toilet right after any high intensity or prolonged exercise. Disgusting right? Sorry, but it was the first thing I noticed. I then noticed that with the same amount of calories consumed, I lost more weight in weeks that I stayed on top of my exercise than when I didn't. I was also more energetic and fit, both of which made me feel good. The more I exercised, the stronger I became and the further I could take my exercise routine.

In my interactions with people trying to lose weight, I have found there are two main categories of people – those who would do anything to lose weight (even take pills and drink strange concoctions) as long as it does not involve exercise, and those who would exercise to any length possible so they can continue to excuse their "all you can eat" lifestyle.

I belonged to the first group, as you can already imagine based on my stories earlier in the book. I would do anything: drink vinegar brews, protein shakes and turmeric concoctions. I even contemplated weight loss pills. Anything but exercise! As a matter of fact, the first time I gave exercise a shot by going on just a 1 mile (1.6km) walk, it was a complete farce: I wore a brand new pair of walking trainers, took photos, and made my husband promise that I would come back to a heavy dish of boiled yam and Nigerian-style fried eggs. Eggs fried the Nigerian way means lots of oil and high calorie additions like corned beef and sardines. I remember coming back from that 1-mile (1.6km) walk and devouring four large yam slices with two eggs fried the Nigerian way. What a waste of time!

If you belong to the second group and believe you can eat as much as you want because you exercise, I hate to burst your bubble. Relying on exercise alone to lose weight is very time consuming, extremely difficult and most probably counterproductive. Here is why...

It takes a deficit of around 7000kcal to lose 1 kilogram (2.2lbs/0.2st.) of fat, although recent research tells us that this may vary by individual depending on age, BMI, gender and other factors. Using my former body weight of 93kg (205lbs/ 14st 9lb) as an example, in order to lose 1kg/2.2lbs (approximately 7000kcal), I will need to do one of these activities:

- Running at 5 mph for 10.5 hours (that is 52.5 miles/84km!)
- Jumping rope for 9.5 hours
- Stair climbing for 12.5 hours
- Swimming for 13 hours
- Brisk walking for 19 hours

If I relied only on exercise, you can imagine how long it would have taken me to lose the 20kg (44lbs/3st 2lb) of weight I lost, also bearing in mind that the above does not take into account any additional calories I would be consuming and piling up at the same time if I didn't change my eating habits. Thank goodness exercise on its own is not the answer to weight loss. There was no way I would have done it.

The good news is that when combined with a healthy balanced diet, you don't need such extremes of exercise to lose weight. Public health experts' advice is that adults between ages 19 and 64 should be physically active daily and engage in at least 150 minutes of moderate intensity physical activity every week. That works out at about 20-25 minutes daily and could be from a variety of activities. I can tell you from personal experience that this level of exercise is more than enough to help you lose weight or maintain a healthy weight if combined with a healthy balanced diet.

Here are the golden rules that worked for me where exercise was concerned:

- **Choose an exercise or fitness activity you can start immediately and sustain.** Ideally, it is something you enjoy and won't get tired of doing after one week. I chose jumping rope (skipping), which is an activity I have loved since primary school. I knew I could sustain it, and it only cost me my skipping rope and nothing more. I also did not have to worry about any gym membership or wait for a marathon event season to get started. I was good to go as soon as my skipping rope was delivered.

- **Take on exercises you can fit around your lifestyle and daily routine.** Although there was a gym in the basement floor at work and my employer offered us subsidised membership, I just couldn't fit it into my schedule. I did school runs before jumping on the train and getting to work on the dot of 9 o'clock at the earliest, or later if there was any train delay. Once it was 5pm, I rushed off so I could get home on time to take on childcare. There was literally no way for me to fit in a visit to the gym. I talked several times about using the gym at work with my work buddies at the time but we just never got around to doing it. Skipping worked perfectly for me as I only did 400 jumps over roughly 10 minutes every weekday morning and a 2.5-mile (4km) walk on Saturday morning.

- **Do whatever works for you.** Skipping was also something I could do in the comfort of my home. All I needed was a little spot in the garden. During winter, I found it hard to go out for my walks or skipping. By the second winter, we had purchased a foldable treadmill thereby making it possible to exercise indoors when it was too cold to go out. I just did what worked for me.

- **Start with baby steps and build on it.** I told you how much of a farce it was on my first attempt at exercising. When I picked up skipping again, I could hardly do 100 jumps without losing my breath and tripping three times in between. By the second week, I was able to do 200, a few weeks later 300, then 400, and sometimes 500 in 10 minutes (including resting breaks). At first, I felt muscle soreness in my legs but that lasted no longer than a few days.

- **Build more physical activity other than your routine exercise into everyday activities.** This could be using the stairs instead of lifts or escalators, walking on local errands rather than driving where possible, parking at the far end of parking lots, running instead of walking up the stairs at home etc. If you use a step counter (and they are even built into your mobile phone nowadays), you will be surprised to see how these seemingly inconsequential activities all add up to the total calories you burn each day.

Workbook Activity: Exercise Planning

Look up different forms of exercises. Select your top five. Think about what you need for each (kit, equipment, clothing, fees/subscriptions, time etc.). In short, count the cost and list what you need to get going.

Now arrange that list in order of their cost from low to high. You may find that your favourite is the highest cost (money and time) to you. That's not a problem. Choose the two you can start the soonest and for which you can get everything you need (exercise kit, accessories, and clothing).

Draw a simple schedule of when you will be carrying out this exercise, time of day and for how long. For example, daily from 6.30 to 6.40am, 5-6pm etc.

Now I need you to start thinking about the forms of exercise you will be taking on. These need to be activities that make you breathe faster and feel warmer to qualify as physical activity. They could be running, brisk walking, skipping, jogging, cycling, swimming, salsa dance, high intensity interval training (HIIT) or online fitness sessions. Don't just leave this open to anything. Decide on specific ones otherwise it is difficult to monitor your progress and you will drop the ball before you have even started. Be sure to seek medical advice first if you have any underlying health issues.

Now that you know everything you need to know for now, there is no need to waste more time. Let's start counting down!

Plan, Cook, Eat and Track

CHAPTER 6

SET YOURSELF
UP TO SUCCEED

This section is all about DOING, and I will be asking you to stop at different points to get things done. Don't rush through this section and don't worry if it takes you days to finish. I would rather you stop, complete assigned tasks and then pick up the book again to continue.

We are now going to start the calorie control lifestyle. I will like to give you a list of the tools you need and how to get them. Get your phone or laptop because you will be downloading, bookmarking and possibly creating a shopping list.

Time to Get Shopping

Now is the time to start shopping your lists beginning with your:

1. **Smart Swap list** especially your newly discovered cupboard ingredients that will be used more often.

2. **Exercise tools, kit, equipment, and clothing.** Remember to begin with the exercise you can start soonest.

3. **Fitness tracker** this could be a Fitbit or any other fitness watch or band. Please note this is optional and there are apps you can download to your phone that will do pretty much the same thing as long as your phone can be on you constantly. I simply downloaded Google Fit onto my phone for free. The advantage of a wearable fitness device is in the name - you can wear it for much longer. Your phone may not always be on you all the time. If you are going paper-based, you can also keep an activity log.

4. **Bathroom scale:** I hope this is already obvious to you. We need a scale if we are going to put our weight in check. You need to make your bathroom scale your friend because it does not lie to you. Once, my husband's visiting pregnant niece asked to check her weight on my scale just before we weighed her luggage. She was not happy

with the weight reading. She thought it was too high and the scale must be faulty. I tried to convince her there was nothing wrong and it is natural to gain some weight during pregnancy but that was just not enough for her. Anyway, we placed her luggage on the scale next and say it weighed 19.1kg *(42lbs/3st)*. When we got to the baggage drop at the airport and placed her luggage on the scale, it read exactly 19.1kg *(42lbs/3st)*. We looked at each other and burst into laughter. "My scale doesn't lie you see," I whispered.

Don't be afraid of your scale. I hear people say you shouldn't check your weight too often if you are trying to lose weight to avoid discouragement. This is nonsense! You need to check your weight daily to see your progress and adjust quickly if progress is slowing. There is no need to be discouraged. You already know the problem and you are doing something about it. You also already know how to solve it. Keep in mind that body weight also fluctuates due to water loss and small changes in the "wrong" direction mean you need to be alert but do not necessarily mean that calorie control is not working. It helps to check your weight about the same time daily for consistency. You cannot manage what you don't measure.

The good news with calorie control is that you will see progress if you stick to your plan. When I started this lifestyle, I told my husband it sounded too good and too simple to be true and I would stop if after two weeks I didn't see a difference in my weight. By the fourth day, although I had lost only 0.2kg *(0.4lb/7.1oz)*, it was lower than my starting weight so I knew if I stuck to it, it would work.

I need you to stop now, pick up your phone or laptop and browse through bathroom scales. You will find everything from basic to multifunctional. Some can measure weight as well as BMI, body fat; bone mass, muscle mass etc. Choose whichever you like and add it to your basket now.

5. **Kitchen scales**: You will need a kitchen scale for weighing your meals and cooking ingredients, especially when trying for the first time to determine the calories in your regular meals. One of the few things that put people off the calorie control lifestyle is weighing. Many people ask me if I weigh every meal. Estimating or "guess-timating" is possible but too open to errors. In the same way, cooking an unfamiliar meal by estimating rather than following a recipe leaves one open to mistakes until one has successfully cooked that meal several times. Achieving my weight goal was so important to me and I wasn't going to base my portion size or calories on estimates or "guess-timates", especially since I have also found that when I love a food so much "guess-timation" plays on my mind

and tends to tell me that more is less. Besides, without knowing the weight and volume of what you are eating and drinking, it is impossible to correctly track your calorie intake. Therefore, my recommendation is to try to be as accurate as you can be when you are in active weight loss mode. There will come a time after you have weighed many meals repeatedly that you can actually tell the amount just by looking. My ask as you start to weigh is to begin taking note of what the weight of your meals equates to in relation to everyday kitchen utensils. For example, through repeated weighing you may learn what one serving spoon of a certain food weighs. This will come in handy when you start to transition from active weight loss to maintenance mode later on.

Your kitchen scale doesn't have to be anything fancy. I still use my Michal mechanical kitchen scale that I bought for just £5 a few years ago, but you could get any type you want, be it digital or mechanical. Can you please pause again, go onto your online shopping to look for a kitchen scale and add that to your basket?

Workbook Activity: Ready - Steady - Go (Shopping list)

Now you know the main things you will need. There will be other minor things to pick up as and when needed. Can you go ahead and complete your shopping list before we move forward?

Shopping done? While we await delivery, let us get your calorie counting system set up and ready to go.

Calorie Tracking System

You will need a way to log and count your calories on an ongoing basis. This can be done manually in hard copy or by using apps. It totally depends on how tech savvy you are or what works for you. I always recommend using apps but we are doing this on your terms and it has to be down to your personal preference.

Hard Copy Journaling System: If you are not technically inclined and would rather log your meals and count your calories manually then there are lots of weight loss diaries and calorie tracking journals that you can choose from online. When selecting, the most important consideration to bear in mind is what you need to record going forward. Ensure your selected diary or journal has enough writing space for documenting your meals and recipes. It should have sections where you can record your weight, including charts, meal plans, exercise logs, and most importantly be able to calculate your total daily calorie intake and any balance or deficits. I recommend the 'Weight Loss Code Breaker – 90 Days Calorie Control Journal'.

You will also need to carry your journal with you everywhere so that you don't miss out on any meal being recorded. I must say that while I would find manual/hard copy tracking difficult, it is not impossible if that is what works best for you.

Calorie Tracking/Weight loss Apps: Now this is my zone. I am highly in favour of using apps or online applications to log calories and track body weight. The beauty of apps, I've found, is that they are very intuitive, user friendly and easy to master even with basic computer skills. You don't need to be tech savvy to work with most. Another good thing is that there are lots of weight loss or calorie tracking apps and you will be spoilt for choice. The Google Play store alone has around 250 weight loss or calorie tracking apps.

The good thing about apps is that they do the heavy lifting for you.

Some of the features you can expect to find on a good weight loss app include:

- A vast food calorie database to select from with an unbelievably large selection of foods that cut across several nationalities and ethnicities. One of my worries starting out was how to find calorie information on traditional Nigerian foods. I was so elated when I found calorie information for egusi, pounded yam, eba, dodo and other favourites on my weight loss app.

- Intuitive adjustment of daily calorie budgets and estimations of the date you will reach your targets based on recorded performance.

- Real-time personalised reports, trends and patterns about what is working or not based on the meals, exercise, and body weight logged.

- The ability to contribute information for foods not currently listed in the calorie database. In essence, some apps are partly community-driven with some information already verified. So if you are unsure, you can go with the information already verified by the developers.

- A platform for logging foods and checking their nutritional information by simply scanning in their barcode. That is one of my favourite features.

- Meal plans, lots of recipes and work out guides that are very useful whether you are new to this way of life or already a pro.

- Ability to link the app to a fitness tool and apps e.g. Fitbit, Google Fit. The app should be able to seamlessly synchronise all your activity information and build it into your daily plan.

- A social aspect enabling users to participate in challenges and share progress with friends.

I hope I have shown you the advantages of an app over a manual system. If it still doesn't seem like your thing, no problem. You will be just fine applying the same principles with a manual system. If yes, you will find there are many options to choose from. While different apps may have different features or be set up in different ways, they mostly follow the same principles so you will be able to apply whatever tips I shared to your chosen app.

A few more things to consider when selecting your app. Always read user reviews, and if available sign up for a free trial. I use the Lose it! app that was recommended to me by a colleague. Some apps have a free basic subscription that offers everything you need to get started. You may want to use the free trial to start, and if you are happy with the app, take it further to the paid subscription to enable you enjoy its full functionality.

Some of the features I mentioned earlier may not be available on free trials or basic subscriptions. If you don't want to download apps onto your phone, most apps will have a web/desktop version you can access on a tablet, laptop or PC.

Remember, the best apps still rely on you logging your meals and exercises daily, so you need to be committed to doing that. The best apps will still not have nutritional information for every single food that exists, so this is where you need to take this information from your back of pack label or the calorie checkers we touched on previously under Smart Swaps.

> **Workbook Activity: Ready or Not?**
> Search the play store/app store or online and choose your preferred app using the information above. Ensure you select a calorie control app. Create your account and download the app. Alternatively, set up your paper-based system.

Set Your Goal

I hope that by now you have started receiving delivery of everything you ordered in the previous chapter. I don't know about you, but I find receiving deliveries of my online shopping exciting. Enjoy it, try it on, take photos, and share with friends. This is all becoming real and you are ready for something life-changing. You will be surprised about how positively life-changing weight loss can be! I am hoping you will enjoy this journey and achieve your goal on time.

As catchy as it might sound to ask you to begin with the end in mind, first you will need to know where you are right now. Hopefully your new scale has arrived! The first thing you need to measure is your **current weight.** Go ahead, stand on the scale and keep your eyes opened. You need to see this weight no matter how bad you think it is. Record your current weight.

Hopefully you know your **height**. If not, get a tape measure and measure. You can simply stand against a wall, get someone to help mark your height, and measure with a tape measure. Otherwise, hop into your local pharmacy or GP and they should be able to help you.

These two pieces of information will be needed to determine your **Body Mass Index** (BMI), which is a good way to tell whether your current body weight is healthy. There is a popular straightforward formula for working out BMI: divide your weight in kilograms by the square of your height in metres. This can be misleading as it does not take your sex, age, ethnicity, or activity level into consideration. I highly recommend the NHS BMI Calculator as it is much more reliable.

Now I need you to go to the NHS BMI calculator *(https:// www.nhs.uk/live-well/healthy-weight/bmi- calculator/)* and use the weight and height you recorded along with other personal information requested to determine your current BMI. Be very honest when doing this as we will be using this information shortly to set your target.

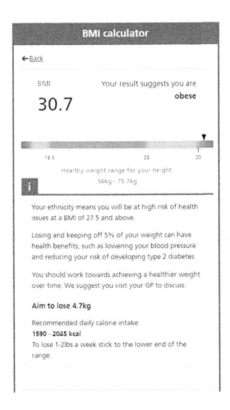

Your BMI should come up as well as a scale showing where you are currently and where your healthy weight range should be. The notes underneath should also indicate the maximum BMI threshold for your ethnicity. The picture you see above was what mine looked like at the start of my weight loss journey. Before this time, I would never have described myself as obese but I got the harsh truth right there.

If you are overweight, you will notice it tells you a suggested amount of weight to lose. If you take that off your current weight and put the difference into the BMI calculator with everything else staying the same, you will find your BMI is reduced but probably not enough to put you in the healthy BMI range. This doesn't mean you are not expected to get into the healthy range. Rather it is an indication that you are expected to lose weight gradually over time (not suddenly) until you get into that healthy range.

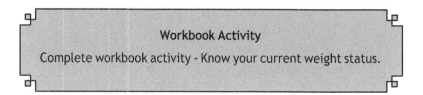

Workbook Activity
Complete workbook activity - Know your current weight status.

Now that you know where you are, you need to set your end goal. Yes, we now need to begin with the end in mind. You have probably heard of SMART goals. SMART stands for

Specific, Measurable, Achievable, Realistic and Time-bound. How does this work in practice?

SPECIFIC: You need to be specific about the target weight required to put you in the healthy BMI range. Based on my BMI result, my healthy weight range is between 56kg *(123lbs/8st 11lb)* and 75.7kg *(166lbs/11st 12lb)*. I needed to lose at least 17.3kg *(38lbs/2st 10lb)* to get to the top end of my healthy BMI. However, setting 75.7kg *(166lbs/11st 12lb)* as my end goal will easily tip me straight into the amber BMI range if I get off track by any chance. So I set myself a target of 73kg *(160lbs/11st 7lb)* allowing a buffer of 2kg *(4.4lbs)* in case I occasionally mess up for whatever reason. You can also decide to set additional goals around other parameters like body fat or activity level. It is totally up to you!

MEASURABLE: Your goal must be measurable. This is where your WHY needs to be converted into a number or other measurable parameter. For instance, if your WHY was to drop two dress sizes, say from UK size 16 to 12, you need to estimate what this corresponds to in measurable terms. For a woman, these will be bust, waist and hip measurements in inches reducing from 41″, 33″ and 43″ respectively to 37″, 28″ and 39″. This means you will need to set a body measurement goal when setting your target. Don't worry if it is not completely accurate, you can always adjust it later if needed.

If your WHY was medical e.g. reducing blood pressure, cholesterol, etc., seek medical advice from your doctor about how much weight you need to lose to achieve your goal. Even when you reach your goal, always consult with a doctor before making changes to your treatment, medication or the frequency of your check-ups.

ACHIEVABLE: Depending on where you are, it may seem unachievable to get back into the healthy weight range. That is a lie and you cannot afford to let that hold you back. Go ahead and set your end goal within the healthy weight range because it is achievable for anyone if you set your heart to it and work towards it. Note that I called it your **END goal** and not your current goal. That is because you can break down that end goal into smaller achievable goals (milestones) and tackle each stage one at a time, but still keeping the END goal in mind. So in my case, even though a BMI of 24-25 will appear to fall within the healthy range, the analysis right below says my ethnicity puts me at an increased risk of health issues with BMI of 23 or more. Having lost my mother to heart condition at 49, coupled with the number of relatives on medication for high blood pressure and diabetes, it was only reasonable that I set my end goal at a weight that puts my BMI below 23. I could control that one risk factor.

My end goal was to get to 73kg *(160lbs/11st 7lb)* but my first milestone was 90kg *(198lbs/14st 2lb)*, then 85kg *(187lb/13st*

5lb), then 80kg *(176lb/12st 8lb).* By the time I got to 80kg *(176lb/12st 8lb),* I was very confident I could do this so I went all the way for the 73kg *(160lbs/11st 7lb)* end goal. Guess what, not only did I meet it, I exceeded it!

Setting my goal to 73kg *(160lbs/11st 7lb)* meant I was able to reduce my BMI from 30.7 to 24 (i.e. from high risk to increased risk for a start). Once that was achieved, my former end goal of 73kg *(160lbs/11st 7lb)* became my new starting point and I started working towards a new end goal to get my weight down to 70kg *(154lbs/11st)* and BMI 23. This would be just fine for me health-wise. God help me with that!

REALISTIC AND REASONABLE: Your end goal needs to be something realistic and reasonable (if I may add my own R), bearing in mind other factors that are peculiar to you. Many failed weight loss attempts are due to unrealistic expectations. Do you honestly think you can lose 10 stones in 10 days? I doubt if anyone can without landing themselves in some serious health problems. This is where you need to ask, "is this goal reachable given the time and resources?" In my case, as much as my look was important to me I wasn't going to set my end goal at 56kg *(123lbs/8st 11lb).* That was my weight 14 years ago when I was underweight. My goal is to be healthy, reduce my health risks and still look very good for my age. It would not make sense to put in all that work only to put myself in another completely new risk category.

So it is important that you read the full analysis below your BMI chart to understand your BMI and the other factors you need to consider in setting your end goal. You may need to go back and try different weight and activity levels in the BMI calculator until you get the weight that corresponds to a healthy BMI for you.

TIME BOUND: There needs to be an endpoint. You should not spend the rest of your life trying to lose weight. At some point, you need to reach your desired weight and move on with your life maintaining it. Besides, it is going to be difficult to set your daily calorie budget if you don't know your target end date.

I cannot emphasise more that you need to lose weight at your own pace. It has to be right for you. Ideally, 0.5kg *(1.1lbs)* weight loss per week is just fine but you could lose up to 1kg *(2.2lbs)* per week. Anything more than that means you will lose muscle mass, which is unhealthy and counterproductive. If using an app, you will get a warning if your target time means you are aiming to lose too much in a short space of time or consuming far less than the minimum recommended calorie intake per day. There is also nothing wrong with losing less than 0.5kg *(1.1lbs)* per week. This journey is more successful when you do it on your terms and at your pace. Weight loss is more sustainable when it is gradual. Never mind what someone else is doing, just mind your own business. I mean that in the nicest possible way! I set myself a six-month target, which meant I wanted to lose just under 1kg (2.2lbs) per week.

Workbook Activities:
Set Your Goal & Set Your Daily Calorie Budget

Once you have decided on your end weight goal, set your target in your app. In my app this was under Goals>Details>Configure>New Program. You will be presented with a range of plans based on weekly weight loss (0.25kg/0.5lbs, 0.5kg/1lbs, 0.75kg/1.5lbs, 1kg/2lbs or maintain current weight) and the corresponding realistic end date. Choose what works for you and you are ready to go!

You should now see your daily calories allowance on the app. As you log your meals, daily exercise, and update your weight as it changes, the app will adjust your daily calorie allowance accordingly.

If you are using a paper-based system, then simply decide how much weight you intend to lose per week and use that to work out when roughly you can meet your target. If your end goal is to lose 4kg/8lbs for example at 1kg/2lbs per week then your target date will be 4 weeks from your start date. Please make sure you write this down in your journal. In order to set your daily calorie budget, you will need to create an account with one of the apps we used above to set your allowance and revert to your manual copy for logging and tracking. You can also use a website such as this one: *https://www.calculator.net/calorie-calculator.html*

You will not be able to benefit from the automatic calorie adjustment using a paper-based system.

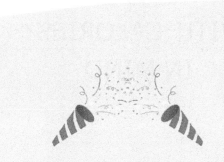

WELL DONE FOR GETTING THIS FAR ON YOUR JOURNEY. A LOT OF PEOPLE GIVE UP BEFORE THEY HAVE EVEN REACHED HERE. FOR GETTING THIS FAR AT ALL, YOU ALREADY DESERVE A MEDAL! WELL DONE!

CHAPTER 7

COOKING WITH CALORIES IN MIND

One of the myths that put people off the calorie control lifestyle is that they need to weigh out every single ingredient every single time they cook a meal. Well, this is not true! We need to bust that myth here and now. We are creatures of habit, and no matter how adventurous, we tend to do the same things repeatedly (especially things that we love, enjoy and seem to work for us). The same goes with cooking: once we know how to cook a meal that we love, most of the time we tend to cook it the same way each time. Even when we give it the occasional twist, the ingredients and core cooking techniques are kept consistent.

You use that same habit in creating and cooking your meals in this new journey you have embarked on. This way, you only need to do the ingredient weighing and calculation of the calorie content of your meals once and save the information for future use.

When cooking your own meals from scratch, you are not likely to have the full calorie information readily at hand. This is a problem, especially for meals from many ethnic cuisines. Even for popular and well-documented recipes, you may have found that some recipe books or websites don't indicate the calories per serving, and if they do, you may be using slightly different ingredients. At some point you will need to work out the calories in the meals that you cook from scratch.

Next time you decide to cook meals from scratch, follow these suggestions:

- **If following a set recipe** where calorie per serving information has been provided; at the end of your cooking, weigh out the entire meal to work out the weight of each serving. If the recipe says it serves four and your cooked meal weighs 1kg (35 oz), you know a serving is 250g (9 oz). I also go further using this information to work out how many calories are in 100g (3.5oz) of that meal. You can then decide if the serving size is right for you and adopt a serving size that will enable you achieve your goal.

- **If cooking without any recipe information,** weigh out all the ingredients you need (remember to switch to your Smart Swap ingredients where applicable). Make a note of the individual ingredient weights on paper or in your app. I definitely recommend you do this with your app as it adds up the calories from each ingredient as you go. If any of your ingredients aren't in the database on your app and you don't have a label to refer to, use the calorie checkers I shared earlier on in the book and as a last resort ask Google. I can assure you there is information online for any ingredient these days. I cook many Nigerian meals and as specialised as some ingredients can be, I have managed to find information for virtually every ingredient; even locust beans! Once you put all your ingredients in the app, it will give you the total calories for that recipe. Cook your meal, weigh out the finished meal and follow the same process described above to decide the right number of servings. For example, if your app says the recipe will deliver 4000kcal and the entire meal weighs 1kg *(35 oz)*, you know this meal will deliver 400kcal per 100g *(3.5 oz)*. Use that to determine your appropriate serving size.

You must then go ahead and save this recipe with the calorie information per serving or per 100g in your app or journal.

That is it, done! Every other time you cook or eat the meal

you do not have to do the weighing rituals all over again, you simply log it by selecting that meal from the database. You may find that you need to do the weigh-to-cook process often at the beginning of your weight loss journey but over time, the frequency drops significantly and you will only need to do it for new meals.

Another myth we need to put to rest is the perception that calorie-controlled meals or recipes designed for weight loss are bland and not delicious. That again is a big fat lie. The secret to success here is to build your meal plans around foods that you love and enjoy. You can also add flavour by using herbs, spices and interesting cooking methods such as smoking food without adding calories. Don't force a food you don't like or enjoy on yourself because it's low calorie. That again is an unsustainable approach. The only exception is if all you love to eat is junk food. You will not be able to lose weight if the basis of your diet is high calorie foods. Create meals to your taste without losing sight of your end goal – balancing nutrients and keeping your calories down.

Don't worry if you are the busy type or haven't been cooking for long.

Personalise recipes and cook meals that fit around your life and work for you. You don't need to be a professional chef to do this. That was exactly the approach I took too.

Without necessarily turning this into a cookbook, I will share some of my favourite quick and easy winning recipes with you. In my book, any recipe that is easy to cook, delicious to eat and consistently keeps me within my calorie budget is a WINNER.

Breakfast Recipes

As a commuting working mum of two, my mornings are planned to the minute and there is no time for messing about. I often only have one and half hours to fit in my devotion time, exercise, putting school pack lunches together, making my breakfast and getting ready for work. Breakfast has to be something I can successfully put together within ten minutes, except Saturdays when I tend to treat my family to a cooked breakfast. That said, I eat with my eyes first so it also has to be appealing but most importantly tasty and filling enough to sustain me through the morning. Despite the rush, I still want to enjoy this meal, which tends to be eaten at my desk as soon as I get into work.

My breakfast recipes are therefore simple but versatile meals that require very little or no cooking at all.

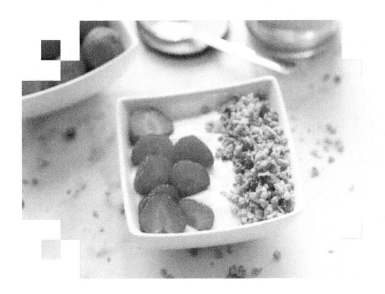

Fruit & Granola Yoghurt Pot

Yoghurt pots are my favourite breakfast by far. They are delicious, filling, low calorie yet balanced and versatile. I make many different versions of this meal. If I was left on a desert island and could only have one food, it would be fat-free Greek yoghurt.

- *Greek-Style fat-free natural yoghurt: 150g / 5oz*
- *Low sugar granola/protein granola: 15g / 0.5oz (optional)*
- *Fresh strawberries: 25g / approx. 1 oz*
- *Honey: 1 teaspoon*

Serves 1 (180kcal)

- Put 150g *(5oz)* fat-free Greek yoghurt into a bowl, sprinkle 15g *(0.5oz)* granola on top of it.
- Dice 25g *(approx. 1oz)* fresh strawberries and layer on the granola. Drizzle 1 teaspoon of honey over it.

Serve with any hot drink of your choice. I have this with green tea or coffee.

This can be made in advance and put in the refrigerator.

Caution: *Resist the temptation to add more granola. Granola is a calorie dense food even when it is low sugar. Over a third of the calories in this recipe come from the 15g (0.5oz) granola.*

Hint: *If you desire more volume, replace granola with an additional 135g yoghurt.*

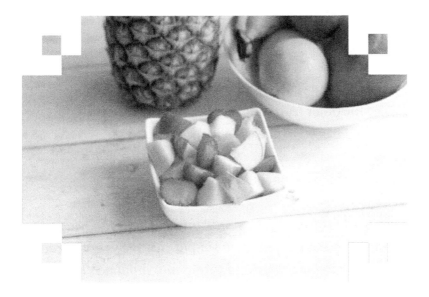

Exotic Fruit Bowl

This breakfast reminds me of home and childhood as it contains two of my favourite fruits growing up: pineapple and mango. Fruit bowls are the superstar breakfast because they are very filling and really low in calories. This recipe, for instance, weighs 300g (10.5 oz) for less than 180 calories. They are versatile and you can try other fruits as you desire. I also use frozen fruit when I am short of fresh fruit.

- *Pineapple: 100g/3.50z*
- *Mango: 50g / 1.80z*
- *Apple: 50g / 1.80z*
- *Pear: 75g / 2.60z*
- *Strawberries: 25g / 0.90z*

Serves 1 (169kcal)

- Wash and peel the pineapple and mango.
- Dice into large cubes and place in a bowl.
- Dice the other fruits and add to the bowl.
- Shake the bowl to get a good mix of the fruits.

Serve with green tea or coffee

Hint: *If using frozen fruits, mix and put into the fridge to defrost for a couple hours. I simply put the frozen fruits together in my lunch box and throw into my lunch bag as I set out for work. It is always ready to eat by the end of my one and a half hour commute.*

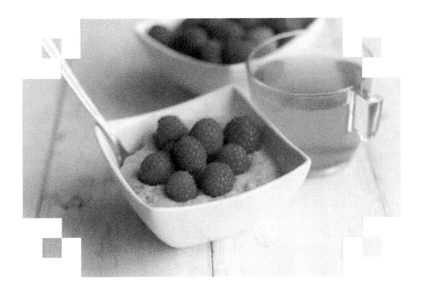

Golden Syrup Oats Porridge Bowl

Growing up and well into adulthood, I never imagined myself eating porridge made of rolled oats. I just disliked any type of lumpy paste. Well, that was until I reluctantly picked up a packet of golden syrup oats sachets while shopping for a self-catering weekend away in 2018. Yes! That was my first shot at eating oats porridge. It was so good and I have not stopped since then.

- *Golden syrup oats porridge: 1 sachet (36g/1.3oz)*
- *Unsweetened Almond Milk: 180ml/6fl oz)*
- *Raspberries: 25g / 0.9oz*

Serves 1 (201kcal)

- Empty the dry oats sachet into a bowl or weigh out 36g (1.3oz) if using a bulk pack of oats.
- Measure out 180ml (6fl oz) of unsweetened almond milk and add to the oats. Stir with a spoon so the oats and milk are well mixed. Cook in the microwave for 2 minutes.
- Take out of the microwave, stir and allow to cool for a minute. Top with raspberries or other desired fruit.

Serve with green tea or coffee.

Hint: *In the absence of a measuring cup for your almond milk, fill your empty sachet to about 1 cm from the top. That is roughly 180ml (6fl oz).*

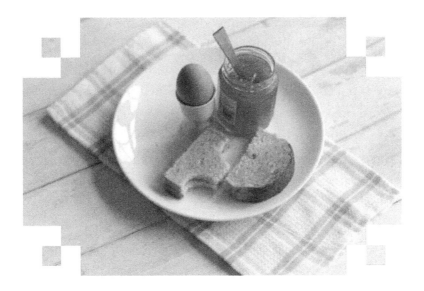

Midweek Toastie Treat

This meal will not sound like a treat to most people but I just enjoy it and always look forward to having it. It is with one of my favourite swaps for white bread – wholemeal or wheat germ bread with calories between 50-64kcal per slice. Toast is not one of those meals that jumps straight to mind when you tell anyone you are losing weight so this for me was a pleasant and welcome surprise.

- *Wheat Germ Bread: 2 slices (29g/1oz per slice)*
- *Apricot Conserve: 15g /0.5oz*
- *Egg: 1*

Serves 1 (227kcal)

- Boil egg for 6 to 8 minutes depending on how you like your egg (soft boiled or hard boiled).
- Once cooked, place in cold water for a couple of minutes to stop it cooking further and make it easier to peel.
- Place bread in the toaster for 1 to 2 minutes or more if you like a crunchier toast.
- Take the bread out of the toaster. Spread your conserve on top of each slice. Peel egg and place beside your toast. That's it.

Serve with green tea, coffee or your favourite hot drink.

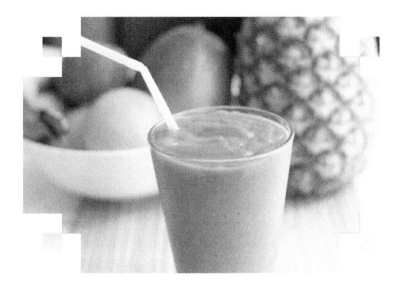

Green Breakfast Smoothie

The smoothie diet was one of the bandwagons I joined because it was trendy but with no understanding of calorie counting. So it did not work for me. I bet it worked for those who knew what they were doing. Now I know better and although I rarely make smoothies anymore, it will be unfair not to let you know you can make smoothies and still keep the calories low by combining the right ingredients in the right proportions.

- *Frozen kale: 40g / 1.4oz*
- *Frozen pineapple chunks: 100g /3.5oz*
- *Fresh ginger: 5g / 0.2oz*
- *Coconut water: 150ml/5fl oz*
- *Banana: 1 small*

Serves 1 (189kcal)

- Place ingredients in a smoothie blender.
- Blend to your desired consistency.
- Pour into glass or smoothie tumbler and enjoy!

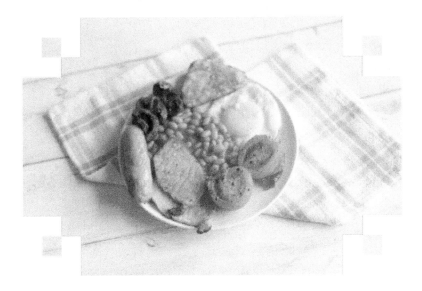

English Breakfast for Less

A girl needs to treat herself too! This is one of my cooked breakfast recipes for weekends or holidays when there is no rush to get out and about. I love my English breakfast and I was intent on keeping it in my diet for fewer calories so I diligently looked for swaps. I was a woman on a mission that morning, intently reading back of pack labels on my local supermarket shelf as if I was going to be taking a test on them. My swaps paid off and my air fryer adds to the magic!

- *Chicken sausages: 2*
- *Hash browns: 2*
- *Eggs: 2*
- *Bacon medallions: 5*

- *Reduced-sugar baked beans: 50g / 1.7oz*
- *Fry light cooking spray: 10 sprays*
- *Cooking salt*
- *Black pepper*

Serves 2 (338kcal per serving)

- Place sausages, bacon and hash browns into the air fryer at 180°C (3560F) for 10 -15 minutes.
- Cooking temperature and time varies when cooking from frozen.
- Check the pack instructions and adjust as necessary.
- For larger batches, consider cooking the hash brown and bacon separately or using the oven.
- Heat a frying pan on low-medium heat.
- Spray cooking spray to cover the base of the pan.
- Fry eggs, seasoning with salt and black pepper.
- Dish all onto a plate and serve with warm baked beans.

Hint: *You can also add other ingredients like tomatoes and mushrooms to this recipe without increasing the calories significantly.*

Main Meals

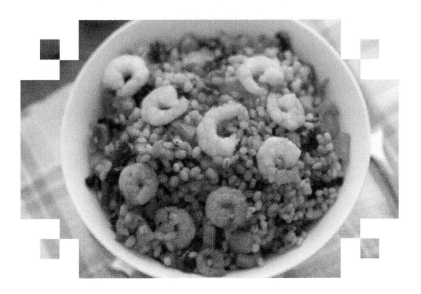

Super Grain, Seafood and Vegetable Stir-fry

Stir-fries are my way of incorporating super grains into my diet and keeping rice in. They are one of my favourite go-to meals for a quick delicious dinner after a long and tiring working day. Stir-fries often deliver a generous portion with lower carbs and a reasonable calorie count. They are versatile and I can put my spicy Nigerian twist on them however I like. In fact, I create so many different versions I might be a self-acclaimed queen of stir-fries.

- *Pearl barley: 250g / 9oz (cooked according to pack instruction)*
- *Olive oil: 4 teaspoons*
- *Vegetable stir-fry mix: 450g /16oz*
- *Garlic: 2 cloves*
- *Onion: 30g / 1oz*
- *King Prawns: 200g / 7oz*
- *Maggi crayfish seasoning cubes: 10g/0.4oz (2 cubes)*
- *(or any choice of seasoning)*
- *Scotch bonnet pepper 1/2 (optional)*
- *(or chilli pepper powder to taste)*
- *Salt (to taste)*
- *Oyster sauce: 2 teaspoons*

Serves 3 (404kcal per serving)

- Heat the oil in a wok or large frying pan on high heat.
- Fry chopped garlic, onion and chilli pepper powder for 1 min.
- Add the prawns and fry for another 2-3 minutes to coat in oil.
- Add the vegetable stir-fry mix and seasoning to taste. Toss to coat in the oil. Fry for another 2-3 minutes.
- Add the cooked pearl barley and mix in thoroughly with the prawns and vegetables.
- Add seasoning, oyster sauce and salt to taste.
- Allow to simmer for about 3 minutes and serve.

Hint: *Use red and yellow pepper, onion, carrot and cabbage if you don't have access to ready-made stir-fry mix. You can try this with several other super grains and they can be pre-cooked too. Sshhhhh!! Can you keep a secret? Shop-bought super grains in microwavable pouches deliver an equally delicious meal. I use them A LOT!*

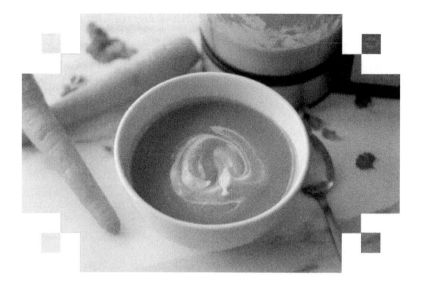

Carrot & Sweet Potato Soup

Soups were my all-time winter favourites even long before I started losing weight. I noticed my weight drops slightly during the winter (pre-Christmas) but it wasn't until I started calorie counting that I realised this might have been the huge number of calories I was cutting from my lunch over winter when I was having soups for lunch almost on a daily basis. They are just so tasty, filling, warming and easy to make, especially when you use a soup maker.

- *Sweet potatoes (cubed): 80g / 3oz*
- *Carrot (diced): 325g / 11oz*
- *Red onion: 25g /0.9oz*

- *Extra virgin olive oil: 2 teaspoons*
- *Reduced-salt chicken stock cube: 1*
- *Fresh or dried coriander (to taste)*
- *Water: 450ml/15fl oz*

Serves 2 (120kcal/serving)

- Put all ingredients in the soup maker or large saucepan. If using fresh coriander, reserve some for serving later.
- Add water to cover the vegetables.
- Put the lid on the soup maker and choose your desired soup texture.
- For this soup, select smooth and switch on. The soup is ready once the soup maker completes its cycle.
- If using a saucepan, simmer until the vegetables are tender then blend.
- If the soup is too thick, add water to get your desired consistency and blend for a few seconds.
- Top with fresh coriander and a dollop of fat-free Greek yoghurt.
- Serve immediately or freeze in single portions for use later.

Hint: *You can also use a slow cooker or regular casserole pan to make the recipe and transfer into a blender to pulse once the vegetables are tender*

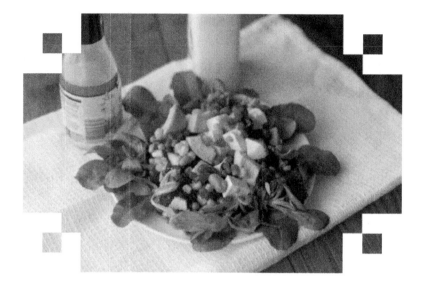

Mixed Bean & Avocado Salad

Salads serve a dual purpose in my diet – as my working lunch or sides to a dinner. I know that salads may make you look like a health geek sometimes, but who cares? Salads give you the freedom to add your own favourite ingredients, any way you like. I don't think there is a right or wrong way when it comes to salads but you need to pay careful attention when adding calorie-dense ingredients like avocado, olives and nuts. The calories soon add up and if care is not taken, you might as well be eating a hamburger and French fries.

- *Bistro-style salad bag: 45g/1.6oz (or any choice of salad leaves)*
- *Black pitted olives: 25g /0.9oz*

- *Sweet corn kernels: 25g /0.9oz*
- *Avocado (flesh): 35g /1.2oz*
- *Light salad cheese: 25g /0.9oz*
- *Mexican bean mix: 30g / 1oz*
- *"Lighter than light" mayonnaise: 10g /0.4oz (or other light salad dressing)*
- *Lemon juice to taste*
- *Black pepper/chilli*

Serves 1 (199kcal)

- Drain Mexican bean mix and rinse under cold running tap (if using frozen, defrost thoroughly and drain).
- Put in a bowl. Cut salad cheese and avocado into cubes. Add to the mixed beans along with the olives and sweet corn.
- To serve, place salad leaves on a plate, spoon your salad on top and drizzle the dressing on it.

Hint: *There are a wide variety of delicious and versatile salad leaves to choose from, such as baby spinach, lettuce, Belgian endive and rocket to name a few.*

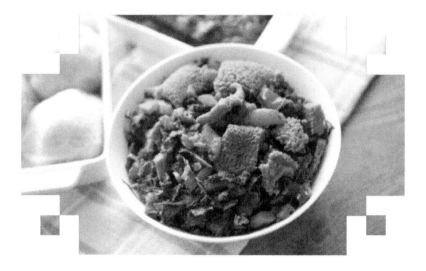

Nigerian Style Vegetable Stew (Efo riro)

Vegetable stews are an integral part of Nigerian cuisine, not just at our parties but part of daily meals in most homes. They are made from various green leafy vegetables (spinach, amaranth, pumpkin leaves, bitter leaf, etc.) and are popularly served as a great accompaniment for staple foods that are often high in carbs. As such, there is a perception that you cannot eat these sorts of meals when you are trying to lose weight. I love Nigerian vegetable stews and would not even think of excluding them from my meals while losing weight. After I started my weight loss journey, it soon became obvious to me that my beloved Nigerian meals could be very healthy if I rethought portion sizes and rebalanced the proportions in my recipes.

When serving traditional Nigerian meals, create a balanced plate by thinking 50-25-25, which stands for 50% vegetable, 25% protein, 25% carbohydrate.

- *Curly kale: 400g /14oz*
- *Palm oil: 3 tablespoons (can be replaced with vegetable oil)*
- *Scotch bonnet (hot) peppers: ½ (to taste)*
- *Onion: 50g /1.8oz*
- *Red Pepper: 200g/7oz*
- *Cherry tomatoes: 100g /3.5oz*
- *Dried crayfish (optional): 10g /0.4oz*
- *Cooked beef tripe: 500g/18oz (also known as shaki)*
- *Locust beans (optional): 2-3 teaspoons (25g/0.9oz)*
- *Maggi crayfish seasoning cube: 20g/0.7oz (2-3 cubes)*
- *Salt*

Serves 5 (215kcal/serving)

- Wash the kale or leafy vegetable of your choice under cold running water and drain. Cut into thin slices about 1 cm wide.
- Fill a medium sized pot with about 1-2 inches of water and bring to boil.
- Place a steam pan in the pot without touching the water. Alternatively use a strainer.

- Fill the steam pan with the sliced vegetables. Cover and allow to steam for 5 minutes until tender.
- Run under cold water quickly for 1 minute to stop the vegetables cooking further. Drain and keep aside.
- Roughly chop onions, tomatoes and pepper into separate bowls. Alternatively, pulse in a blender for a few seconds. You want a rough and chunky mix.
- Heat oil in a pan until very hot. Add some of the chopped onion and cook for 1-2 minutes, then add the rough chopped or blended tomato and pepper mix and the remaining onion.
- Cook on moderate heat for 5 minutes. If using diced vegetables, add a small amount of water to stop sauce from burning.
- Add locust beans, dried crayfish, seasoning and stir to mix into the sauce.
- Cut or dice the cooked offal into desired size. Add into the stew and stir. Add salt to taste. Cover, reduce heat and cook for a further 5 minutes.
- Put the steamed kale in and stir until well coated with the meat stew. Allow to simmer for 2-3 minutes. Remove from heat.

Serve with grilled fish, turkey, chicken or lean beef.

Sides: 125-200g (4.4 - 7oz) rice or other traditional Nigerian starchy staples (popularly referred to as 'solids') depending on calorie allowance.

105

Hints: *This recipe delivers 108kcal per 100g (3.50z) of vegetable stew and steaming helps lock in flavour and nutrients better than blanching with hot water.*

Do not exceed 200g (7oz) of starchy sides as these are energy dense. Contrary to how this is served traditionally, the vegetable stew is the main meal and the starchy 'solids' or rice is your side so should be significantly less.

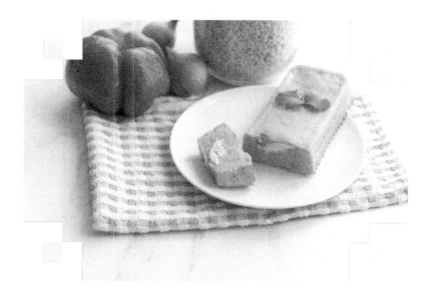

Nigerian Steamed Bean Pudding (moin moin)

Growing up, moin moin was my Dad's favourite meal and Mum used to joke that any woman who wants to snatch her man must first be excellent at making moin moin. Thankfully, Grandma ran a street food business that specialised in moin moin so all her daughters, my mum inclusive, are pros at making moin moin. You will find moin moin served as an accompaniment in Nigerian parties but it can be a main meal on its own that is filling, delicious, rich in protein and surprisingly not calorie dense. The only thing I disliked about moin moin growing up was peeling the beans. Now I save myself the hassle by using peeled beans. It delivers the exact same result so don't be precious about peeling your own beans.

- *Peeled black eyed beans or brown beans: 950g / 34oz*
- *Large red pepper: 2*
- *Fresh scotch bonnet (hot) pepper: 2*
- *Onion: 1*
- *Dried Crayfish: 15g /0.5oz*
- *Hardboiled egg: 4*
- *Vegetable oil: 4 tablespoons*
- *Homemade chicken/beef stock: 200ml/6.7fl oz*
- *Maggi chicken/crayfish seasoning cube: 40g /1.4oz*
- *Salt (to taste)*
- *Water: 1.5l*
- *Small aluminium foil plates with lids (for cooking)*

Serves 10 (142kcal/serving)

- Put peeled beans in a bowl, cover with water and leave to soak for 1-2 hours. In the meantime, boil eggs, peel and slice into small pieces (ideally 2-4 per egg). Set aside for use later. Chop peppers and onion.
- Once the beans have been soaked, blend in a food processor in small batches with the stock, peppers and onion into a smooth thick paste. Add water as you blend if needed to make the blender work better. The paste needs to be very smooth with no bean granules.
- Pour beans paste into a mixing bowl. Stir and slowly add the remaining water until you get a lighter puree consistency.

I use about 1 litre of water and stock altogether (including water added during blending) to get the consistency right. If you have more homemade chicken/beef stock, you can use it to replace some of the water.

- Add seasoning cube, crayfish and vegetable oil. Keep stirring to mix in all the ingredients.
- Use a large serving spoon or ladle to portion mixture into individual aluminum foil plates and add eggs onto each. Cover each plate with the lid securely.
- Put a large pot on the cooker and add water up to about 3 inches. Arrange moin moin in the pot and cover to cook. Check regularly and add water as and when needed to stop the *moin moin* from burning. Cook on moderate heat for 45 minutes to 1 hour.
- To check if your *moin moin* is cooked, open and put a skewer through the *moin moin*. Your moin moin is ready if the skewer comes out clean. If not, cover and continue cooking for longer. The cooking time for *moin moin* depends on the type of container, quantity and the size of your cooking pot.
- Once cooked, remove from heat, take *moin moin* out of the pot or leave the pot slightly opened to let out the steam and allow moin moin to cool.

To serve: Remove the foil lid and turn upside down on to a plate. The moin moin should come out neatly.

Moin moin can be enjoyed alone or with other sides.

Hint: *You can use other containers instead of foil plates or traditional moin moin leaves; just grease them before putting in the moin moin paste. You can also use other garnishes such as smoked fish and cooked lean mince in addition to or in place of egg. Moin moin cooks faster if arranged in the pot in alternating layers to allow steam to reach each container quicker.*

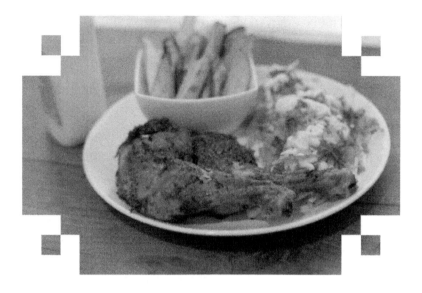

Guilt-free chicken & chips

My kids love chicken & chips so much it has become one of their favourite mid-week lunches once they get back from school. The truth is, my husband and I have also come to love this as a lazy Saturday lunch or dinner. As such, chunky steak-cut chips are a regular part of our grocery shopping list. Chicken & chips is one meal that highlights our personal differences as a family. Hubby and I like it with mayonnaise, our daughter with ketchup and our son with barbecue sauce. I still enjoy guilt-free chicken & chips, having replaced most of the ingredients with my smart swaps to keep calories in check.

- *Sweet potatoes: 200g/7oz*
- *Parsnips: 150g /5oz*
- *Chicken Legs: 2 (200g/7oz roasted)*
- *Fry light cooking spray*
- *Thyme*
- *Rosemary*
- *Salt*
- *Black Pepper*
- *Cajun/Fajita Spice*
- *Lighter-than-light mayonnaise: 15g/0.50z*

Serves 2 (350kcal/serving)

- Season chicken with salt, Cajun spice and rosemary. Marinate in a refrigerator for 1-2 hours.
- Preheat the oven or air fryer to 180ºC (3560F). Place seasoned chicken on a lined tray into the oven or directly into the air fryer. Allow to cook for 30 minutes.
- While chicken cooks in the oven or air fryer, wash and cut parsnips and sweet potatoes (with or without skin) into rectangular slices similar to steak cut chips.
- Place in a bowl. Spray some oil over the chips (10-20 sprays). Add salt, thyme and black pepper. Shake together to evenly coat chips with the oil and seasoning.
- If using an oven, place chips on a lined oven tray and bake at the same temperature for 15-20 minutes.

- If using an air fryer, fry at the same temperature for 15-20 minutes.

Serve with lighter-than-light mayonnaise (or desired low-calorie sauce) and salad.

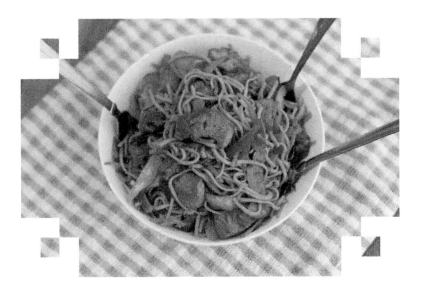

Stir-fried pork noodles

Pork never crossed my mind as one of the meats I could still have in my diet. Thanks to a TV ad comparing it to chicken breast, I dug deeper and found out that pork fillet (also known as tenderloin) is very lean. This could only be great news for a meat lover like myself! Of course, it went straight into my diet and first into this deliciously filling meal that also doubles as a family favourite.

- *Lean Pork fillet (diced): 425g/15oz*
- *Egg noodles: 100g/3.5oz*
- *Stir-fry vegetable mix: 300g /11oz*
- *Olive oil: 1½ tablespoons*

- *Reduced salt soy sauce: 1 tablespoon*
- *Seasoning cubes: 3 (15g/0.5oz)*
- *Ginger: 2cm, grated*
- *Garlic: 2 cloves*
- *Chilli powder (to taste)*
- *Salt (optional)*

Serves 3 (440kcal/serving)

- Cook egg noodles in line with pack instruction. Drain in a colander and keep aside.
- Chop garlic finely. Heat a wok or frying pan on high heat. Add oil and part of the garlic to the hot pan at the same time. Adding garlic before oil heats up allows it to infuse flavour into the oil rather than being burnt instantly.
- Add the rest of the garlic and diced pork and fry for 3-4 minutes until it has browned, turning it so that it cooks evenly.
- Add ginger and stir-fry vegetable mix to the meat and fry together for a further 2-3 minutes while continuously stirring. Add seasoning and dried chilli powder.
- Add noodles to the meat and vegetable stir-fry. Stir in for even distribution of meat and vegetables. Drizzle soy sauce and stir in to evenly coat everything in the pan. Add salt (if needed).
- Allow to cook for about 2 minutes and serve immediately.

Hint: *I use shop bought premixed stir-fry vegetables but you can put yours together with readily available vegetables like cabbage, carrot, red pepper and red onion. It is even nicer if you have bean sprout and mangetout to add to your vegetable mix.*

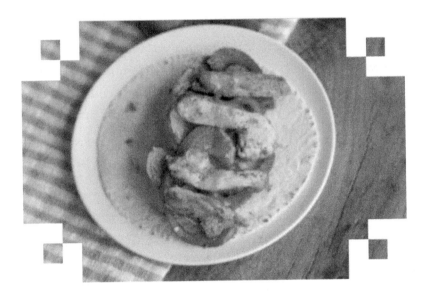

Chicken Wrap

Taking control of calories in my midweek lunches while working was one of my concerns when I started my weight loss journey. Wraps are very versatile as you can wrap up many different combinations of protein, vegetables and a delicious dressing. This recipe uses chicken but I have used beef trimmings, turkey slices, avocado, prawns etc. Name it and you can wrap it!

- *Skinless chicken breast fillet: 100g /3.5oz*
- *Red pepper: 10g/0.4oz*
- *Mini tortilla wrap: 1*
- *Reduced salt soy sauce: 1 teaspoon*

- *Lettuce: 21g/0.7oz*
- *Peri-peri sauce (or any other sauce of choice): 1 teaspoon*
- *Salt (optional)*
- *Black pepper*
- *Chilli (optional)*
- *Cooking spray*

Serves 1 (209kcal/ serving)

- Cut chicken breast fillet into thick slices. Season with salt, black pepper and/or chilli.
- Add cooking spray to a frying pan on medium to high heat. Fry the seasoned chicken slices for 3-4 minutes, turning it so both sides cook evenly.
- Add sliced red pepper and stir-fry for a further 2 minutes. Drizzle on the soy sauce. Stir in and simmer for 1 minute.
- Remove from heat ensuring your chicken has cooked through. Cooking time may vary with the thickness of your slices.
- Warm tortilla wrap in line with pack instruction or use straight from the pack.
- Place tortilla wrap on a flat surface; lay a lettuce leaf on the wrap with the hollow side facing up.
- Fill the lettuce with your chicken mix. Drizzle peri-peri sauce or your preferred sauce over it.
- Wrap and enjoy!

YEMI FADIPE

Hint: *The protein filling can be made in advance for reheating and wrapping when it is ready to be served*

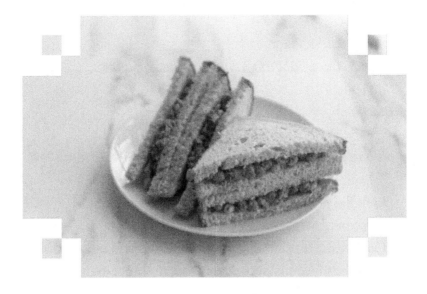

Sardine Sandwich

This recipe will not make sense to a regular sandwich consumer but I am not one of the regulars. I cannot stand tuna and don't like leaves with my bread. It's odd. Right?

So as you would expect, I made mine up with one of my favourite fish and two veggies I could eat for life – peas and sweetcorn. Don't ask what I was thinking putting this together, just try it! It is one of my quickest midweek lunch mash ups for work.

- *Wholemeal or wheat germ bread 4 slices (29g/1oz per slice)*
- *Sardines: 1 can*

- *Green peas: 25g /0.9oz*
- *Sweet corn: 25g/0.9oz*
- *Lighter-than-light mayonnaise: 2 teaspoons*
- *Salt (pinch)*
- *Black pepper*

Serves 2 (216kcal/serving)

- Drain the sardines from the can and place in a small bowl. Each can contains roughly 3 fillets.
- Mash with a fork. Add salt, pepper, peas and sweet corn. Mix in the mayonnaise to evenly coat the other ingredients.
- Spread on a slice of bread. Cover with the second slice and cut into rectangular or diagonal shaped sandwiches.

These are all quick, easy and basic recipes to show you that cooking healthy meals does not have to be complicated, especially for people who don't have the time or don't particularly enjoy cooking. If you are the budding chef type or like me just enjoy cooking, then by all means go ahead, experiment with various ingredients and try out your skills with more elaborate recipes.

The message is whether gourmet or basic, healthy cooking is doable with any level of cooking proficiency and any ethnic cuisine as long as you cook with calories in mind.

Workbook Activity:

Complete workbook activity - Create Your Recipe Cards

CHAPTER 8

MEAL PLANNING

Now that you know your daily calorie target, permit me to introduce you to a new way of seeing it. Just as cash is king in the world of business, calorie is king in the world of weight management. Your daily calorie budget is your currency and you need to treat it the way you treat your money.

Let us draw a few analogies:

You always want to get good value for money. Yes, you also need to get good value for your calories. Will you spend 588kcal on 100g (3.5oz) of honey-roasted peanuts when the same amount of calories can get you a delicious, filling and satisfying dinner? This is not some random example. I once did it without checking the back of pack label before digging into the snack. Oops! Half of my calorie budget for the day was gone just like that in a moment of uncontrolled snacking. I was so annoyed I wrote the retailer to complain about the label being misleading – calling the product honey-roasted when it is actually drowning in sugar. Another way to look at this is considering the nutritional value of your choices. If presented with crisps and nuts at the same calories, then your criteria for choosing becomes the nutritional value of nuts over crisps. This does not detract from the fact that you can also gain weight eating healthy snacks if you consistently exceed your target so you should still keep an eye on the calorie count especially with healthy but calorie dense foods.

You want to get more for less with your money. This is intertwined with getting value for your money and this is where your smart swaps come in. Why get one slice of white bread for 120kcal when the same amount of calories can get me two slices of equally tasty Weight Watchers medium white bread and still give me a balance of 20kcal?

You need to stretch your calorie allowance to get more food for less calories, and one of the ways to do this is to incorporate more vegetables. They are filling, mostly less calorie-dense and deliver more volume for fewer calories compared to other food groups.

Money spent here cannot be spent there. If you have not heard this before it means the more money spent on one thing, the less money will be available to spend on something else. This is a useful concept in money management that you need to bring with you on your weight loss journey. Just say you have 1000kcal to spend today and you spend 588kcal on honey-roasted peanuts like me. The 588kcal is spent, it is gone, and you do not have it again for that day. Now you are left with only 412kcal to cover your breakfast, lunch and dinner. Not sure how I could fare with that!

You may not be able to get spent money back but you can make more money. It is harder to make money than to spend it. There is a saying in my language that "money resides in the mouth of lions." In essence, it takes the conscientious, bold and courageous to get it out. In the same light, you can also raise your daily calorie allowance on any given day by stepping up your exercise and activity level. For instance, my app awards me a bonus of 245kcal on days that I walk 7750 steps and a bonus of 100kcal when I do my ten minutes of skipping (jumping rope). This gets added to my calorie allowance for the day, which means I can get more food. Don't worry, the app is clever and it is not giving you back all the calories you burnt from exercising. You will not be able to lose weight if that happens! Far more calories have been burnt walking 7750 steps or doing 400 to 500 skips in ten minutes.

Here comes the only point of difference between money and your daily calorie budget:

You cannot carry over your balance from the previous day! Any unspent calories for the day are gone. Your balance resets the next day. It is important that you respect this golden rule otherwise your weight won't move an inch. There is a reason why "daily" is included when calories and nutrients are mentioned. Have you thought about it? Recommended Daily Intake, Guidance Daily Allowance, Daily Calorie Intake, Recommended Daily Amount, etc.

It is a daily affair. No carryovers.

30-Day Calorie Control Meal Journal
Rather than give you a meal plan prescribing what to eat and what not, in this section I have decided to share my meal journal with you, showing a realistic and live application of the calorie control approach based on my actual diary when I was in active weight loss mode.

I decided not to force a meal plan down your throat with meals you may not like, never eat or have never heard of and ingredients that may not be readily available to you. My intention is to show you that you can do this on your own terms as I did. You can do it with any ethnic cuisine you are familiar with and ingredients that are available to you. I hope you can learn some techniques that you can use effectively during your calorie control journey.

These 30 days have been selected randomly from the six months when I was actively in weight loss mode and shed 20kg/44lbs/3st 2lbs (from 93kg (205lbs/14st 9lbs) in April to 73kg (160lbs/11st 6lbs) in October).

In this 30-day journal, you will see what those days looked like in terms of my targets, meals, exercise, and activity level and how my weight decreased gradually. The goal is for you to understand how all those factors work together to help you achieve your weight loss goal when properly executed.

You can then use this as a template to build your own meal plan.

Date	Body weight (kg/ibs)	Daily calorie budget (kcal)	Breakfast	Lunch	Dinner	Snacks & drinks	Planned Exercise	Steps count-ed	Calorie balance / deficit (kcal)	Notes
23-Apr	93kg 205lbs	1315	Banana & almond smoothie, green tea (365kcal)	Chicken salad with mayo, low sugar lemonade (363kcal)	Wholegrain & quinoa seafood & vegetable stir-fry (484kcal)	Coffee with skimmed milk (no sugar, 12kcal) Pecan nuts 76g (559kcal)	10 mins Skipping 10 mins low impact aerobics (-176kcal)	141	293	Not a great start. Poor selection of snack robbed me of nearly half my target and pushed me into deficit.
03-May	87.8kg 193.5lbs	1288	Fat-free natural yoghurt topped with granola and honey (213kcal)	Black bean & avocado salad (105kcal)	Quinoa & mung bean pepper stir fry with grilled hake fish (573kcal)	Oatcakes with almond butter (153kcal), coffee with skimmed milk (no sugar, 11kcal)		1680	232	Missed exercise but calorie allowance was managed better. Weight starting to decrease.

Date	Body weight (kg/lbs)	Daily calorie budget (kcal)	Breakfast	Lunch	Dinner	Snacks & drinks	Planned Exercise	Steps counted	Calorie balance / deficit (kcal)	Notes
04-May	91.1kg 200.8lbs	1288	Fat-free Greek yoghurt topped with granola and honey (352kcal)	Seeded wholemeal turkey sandwich (296kcal)	Pounded yam with egusi soup and cow skin (733kcal)	Coffee with skimmed milk (no sugar, 11kcal)	5 mins skipping (-72kcal)	1346	32	Discovered granola and seeded breads are calorie-dense. Smart Swap research begins in earnest.
07-May	89.7kg 197.7lbs	1267	Banana & pineapple cake, black tea with skimmed milk (366kcal)	Nigerian vegetable stew with quinoa & mung beans, diet coke (345kcal)	Nigerian meat pie (504kcal)	Diet coke (2kcal), gari (cassava flour) and peanuts (274kcal)	Morning walk (2.6miles, 4699 steps)	3507 (-245 kcal)*	4	Yay! I exceeded my steps target today and got a bonus. My love for gari caught up with me today and I couldn't resist it. It borders between snack and a meal, either way my bonus paid for it. *bonus from total steps

129

Date	Body weight (kg/ibs)	Daily calorie budget (kcal)	Breakfast	Lunch	Dinner	Snacks & drinks	Planned Exercise	Steps count-ed	Calorie balance / deficit (kcal)	Notes
13-May	88.7kg 195.5lbs	1253	Fasting morning	Nigerian vegetable stew with pounded yam, grilled hake (398kcal)	Nigerian meat pie, hot chocolate with skimmed milk (677kcal)	Mint tea (4 kcal), snack crackers (92kcal)				I finally nailed the correct portion size for my heavy Nigerian pounded yam. No exercise today. I find it hard on mornings when I am fasting. This fasting is religious and not for dieting.
28-May	86.7kg 191lbs	1224	Fat-free Greek yoghurt topped with blueberries, granola and honey (250kcal)	Nigerian jollof rice with oven baked chicken thigh and coleslaw (517kcal)	Grilled lamb with corn on cob (399kcal)	Black tea w/skimmed milk (11kcal), shortbread cookies (100kcal)	Morning walk (2.6miles, 4699 steps)	3446 (-236 kcal)*	183	Took the opportunity of the bank holiday to ramp up my steps today. It paid off and I rewarded myself with my best cookies in the whole wide world. *bonus from total steps

Date	Body weight (kg/ibs)	Daily calorie budget (kcal)	Breakfast	Lunch	Dinner	Snacks & drinks	Planned Exercise	Steps counted	Calorie balance / deficit (kcal)	Notes
10-Jun	84.8kg 186.9ibs	1189	Fat-free Greek yoghurt topped with blueberries, granola and honey (169kcal)	Nigerian vegetable stew with pounded yam, air fried turkey (766kcal)	Wholemeal banana & almond butter sandwich, reduced fat hot chocolate with skimmed milk (330kcal)	Shortbread cookies (114kcal)	Morning walk (2.6miles, 4699 steps)	3799 (-240 kcal)*	52	Yay! My 85kg milestone achieved! Another weekend, another bonus thanks to being able to do my planned walk in addition to household errands. *bonus from total steps
13-Jun	84.8kg 186.9ibs	1189	Carrot, spinach and berry smoothie (259kcal)	Wholemeal banana & peanut butter sandwich (193kcal)	Nigerian okra vegetable stew with amala (yam flour) (459kcal)	Kellogg's chocolate & raspberry cereal bar (86kcal)	6 mins skipping (-96kcal)	1113	289	Discovered peanut butter has fewer calories than almond butter and I'm starting to enjoy my new swap.

Date	Body weight (kg/lbs)	Daily calorie budget (kcal)	Breakfast	Lunch	Dinner	Snacks & drinks	Planned Exercise	Steps count-ed	Calorie balance / deficit (kcal)	Notes
15-Jun	84.6kg 186.5lbs	1186	Hardboiled egg, tea with skimmed milk (81kcal)	Grilled chicken and asparagus salad (299kcal)	Bulgur wheat, quinoa and wholegrains, spinach, vegetable stew, air fried turkey (585kcal)	Oatcakes with peanut butter (74 kcal), tea with skimmed milk (no sugar, 11kcal), shortbread cookies (171kcal)	6 mins skipping (-96kcal)	499	96	Too little breakfast today meant I ended up snacking up more, and I am still not over my shortbread addiction.
19-Jun	84.2kg 185.6lbs	1180	Pineapple, banana and spirulina smoothie (222kcal)	Wholemeal banana & peanut butter sandwich (182kcal)	Chicken and baked sweet potatoes with homemade coleslaw (471kcal)	Cashew nuts (146kcal), peanuts (148kcal)	6 mins skipping (-95kcal)	840	107	Experimenting with nuts again today. Nuts have been my undoing on several occasions now but it seems I am closer to getting the right portion size. 25 g of each today looked really small

Date	Body weight (kg/lbs)	Daily calorie budget (kcal)	Breakfast	Lunch	Dinner	Snacks & drinks	Planned Exercise	Steps count-ed	Calorie balance / deficit (kcal)	Notes
28-Jun	83.1kg 183.2lbs	1164	Fat-free Greek yoghurt topped with strawberries , granola and honey (202kcal)	Avocado & mixed peppers wrap (275kcal)	Nigerian spinach stew, red beans and spicy Mexican rice, air fried turkey (504kcal)	Sweet chilli plantain chips (170kcal) Coffee w skimmed (11kcal) Tea w skimmed milk (11kcal)	6 mins skipping (-94kcal)	764	84	Got everything happening on my dinner plate tonight, a fusion of different ethnic cuisines or just putting leftovers together but it actually came together nicely.
										but maybe nuts are not made for bulk consumption as I used to eat them.

Date	Body weight (kg/lbs)	Daily calorie budget (kcal)	Breakfast	Lunch	Dinner	Snacks & drinks	Planned Exercise	Steps counted	Calorie balance / deficit (kcal)	Notes
09-Jul	81.1kg 178.8lbs	1136	Fat-free Greek yoghurt topped with fresh mixed berries, granola and honey (158kcal)	Avocado salad (318kcal)	Nigerian red beans, sweet potato and chicken (537kcal)	Tea with skimmed milk (11kcal)		4522	112	
12-Jul	80.6kg 177.7lbs	1128	Fat-free Greek yoghurt topped with fresh mixed	Wholemeal egg sandwich (202 kcal)	Rice and lentils with Nigerian spinach stew, garnished	Crackers (92kcal), green tea (0kcal)	8 mins skipping (-122kcal)	1795	471	I have a significant number of calories outstanding today. Seems like a winning performance but today's calorie intake is too low for comfort.

Date	Body weight (kg/lbs)	Daily calorie budget (kcal)	Breakfast	Lunch	Dinner	Snacks & drinks	Planned Exercise	Steps counted	Calorie balance / deficit (kcal)	Notes
			berries, granola and honey (185kcal)		with turkey gizzard & beef tripe (300kcal)					
13-Jul	81.2kg 179lbs	1137	Fat-free Greek yoghurt topped with fresh mixed berries, granola and honey (183kcal)	Chicken salad (216kcal)	not logged	not logged	Morning walk (2.6 miles, 4699 steps)	1406		Attending couple's weekend away with hubby this weekend starting tonight until Sunday. Last thing on my mind at a 4 star romantic retreat is counting calories. Sorry weight loss app. We'll resume business as usual on Monday
14-Jul								261		

Date	Body weight (kg/lbs)	Daily calorie budget (kcal)	Breakfast	Lunch	Dinner	Snacks & drinks	Planned Exercise	Steps count-ed	Calorie balance / deficit (kcal)	Notes
18-Jul	81.2kg 179lbs	1137	Fat-free Greek yoghurt topped with strawberries, granola and honey (231kcal)	Mexican prawn Salad (183kcal)	Super seed mix, spinach stew with grilled hake & panmo (beef skin) (594kcal)	Crackers (92kcal) Tea w skimmed milk (11kcal), coffee with skimmed milk (11kcal)	8 mins skipping (-107kcal)	131	122	Back to life, back to reality!
24-Jul	79.9kg 176lbs	1130	Wholemeal banana & peanut butter sandwich (207kcal)	Tomato & mozzarella salad (312kcal)	Wholegrain bulgur wheat & quinoa stir-fry served with moin moin & grilled hake (477kcal)	Crackers (115 kcal), tea with skimmed milk (11kcal), coffee with skimmed milk (11kcal)	7 mins skipping (-106kcal)	545	103	

Date	Body weight (kg/lbs)	Daily calorie budget (kcal)	Breakfast	Lunch	Dinner	Snacks & drinks	Planned Exercise	Steps count-ed	Calorie balance / deficit (kcal)	Notes
23-Aug	78.3kg 172.6lbs							9381 (-247 kcal)		Never thought we did these many steps walking across airports. Summer vacation week in Croatia starts today. Impossible to count calories but whilst I am enjoying every plate this week I am making the effort to visit the gym to treadmill for 30 minutes daily
29-Aug	78.6kg 173.3lbs	1111	Fat-free Greek yoghurt topped with blueberries,	Salmon and bean salad (180kcal)	Mixed vegetable quinoa & mung bean stir-fry,	Oreo cookie (70kcal), banana & peanut (201kcal), tea w	8 mins skipping (-104kcal)	5362	13	Holiday is over and I have only added 0.3kg. That for me is success! Now I need to get back in the groove. I struggled a

Date	Body weight (kg/ibs)	Daily calorie budget (kcal)	Breakfast	Lunch	Dinner	Snacks & drinks	Planned Exercise	Steps count-ed	Calorie balance / deficit (kcal)	Notes
			granola and honey (220kcal)		grilled hake (534kcal)	skimmed milk (11kcal), coffee w skimmed milk (11kcal)				little today and snacked more. Holiday hangover!
01-Sep	76.2kg 167.9lbs	1076	Pancake topped with honey, low fat hot chocolate (198kcal)	Nigerian red beans (324kcal)	Baked sweet potato and chicken (439kcal)	Crackers (69kcal), tea with skimmed milk (11kcal)	Morning walk (2.6 miles /4km 4699 steps)	2446	35	Experimented making pancakes from wholemeal wheat flour today.
04-Sep	76.2kg 167.9lbs	1076	Fruit bowl 177kcal)	Wholemeal banana & peanut butter	7 rice & grains oriental stir-fry, air	Tea with skimmed milk (11kcal), coffee	7 mins skipping (101kcal)	3755	76	I love this 7 rice & grains microwave rice. Cheap, easy, convenient, 2 minute cook time and

Date	Body weight (kg/lbs)	Daily calorie budget (kcal)	Breakfast	Lunch	Dinner	Snacks & drinks	Planned Exercise	Steps counted	Calorie balance / deficit (kcal)	Notes
				sandwich (247kcal)	fried turkey (655kcal)	with skimmed milk (11kcal)				low calories. What more can I ask for in my stir-fry?
05-Sep	76.2kg 167.9lbs	1076	Oatcakes, peanut butter (206kcal)	Prawn cocktail sandwich, tuna sandwich, deep fried chips (379kcal)	7 rice & grains oriental stir-fry, grilled hake (577kcal)		8 mins skipping (101kcal)	3490	15	Working lunch with colleagues today. Calories logged was a guess-timate.
15-Sep	77.6kg 171lbs	1096	Breakfast omelette (621kcal)	Nigerian moin moin (150kcal)	Fried plantain with	Low fat hot chocolate (39kcal)		4492	1	Took my son out to breakfast today to mark the end of 11+ exam

Date	Body weight (kg/lbs)	Daily calorie budget (kcal)	Breakfast	Lunch	Dinner	Snacks & drinks	Planned Exercise	Steps count-ed	Calorie balance / deficit (kcal)	Notes
					vegetable stew and beef tripe (285kcal)					season. Luckily, the café had calorie information on the menu. With breakfast taking half of my calorie allowance, I need to adjust lunch and dinner to keep within target.
17-Sep	76.8kg 169.3lbs	1085	Fat-free Greek yoghurt topped with strawberries, granola and honey (208kcal)	Prawn & avocado salad (183kcal)	7 rice & grains beef stir-fry, grilled turkey (564kcal)	Crackers (69kcal), low fat hot chocolate (39kcal), tea with skimmed milk(11kcal)	7 mins skipping (102kcal)	1971	2	

Date	Body weight (kg/lbs)	Daily calorie budget (kcal)	Breakfast	Lunch	Dinner	Snacks & drinks	Planned Exercise	Steps count-ed	Calorie balance / deficit (kcal)	Notes
						, coffee with skimmed milk (11kcal)				
30-Sep	75.4kg 166.2lbs	1065	Banana, coffee w skimmed milk (132kcal)	Nigerian vegetable stew w Pounded yam, grilled hake (694kcal)	Baked sweet potato & chicken (252kcal)			440	-13	It's always a rush to get to church (about 50 miles /80km away) on Sunday mornings, so there is no remote chance of fitting in planned morning exercise. I need to think of fitting this into Sunday evenings.
02-Oct	75kg 165.3lbs	1059	Fat-free Greek yoghurt topped with	Wholemeal egg sandwich (195kcal)	Eba with egusi stew and beef tripe	Tea & coffee with unsweetened almond	7 mins skipping (-99kcal)	1421	-16	Food-wise it was a good day but my budget has been adjusted again with my new weight, so I need to adjust.

Date	Body weight (kg/lbs)	Daily calorie budget (kcal)	Breakfast	Lunch	Dinner	Snacks & drinks	Planned Exercise	Steps count-ed	Calorie balance / deficit (kcal)	Notes
			strawberries, protein granola and honey (161kcal)		(697kcal)	milk (6kcal), crackers (115kcal)				
03-Oct	74.8kg 164.9lbs	1056	Fasting morning	Moin moin, brown rice with egusi soup and beef tripe (256kcal)	Mixed vegetable, bulgur wheat and quinoa prawn stir-fry (442kcal)	Banana & peanuts (342kcal), coffee with unsweetened almond milk (6kcal)		1092	10	Banana with peanuts is one of my odd but favourite snacks. Not sure what difference fasting made today as I still ended up eating almost 3 square meals. Good news though, I found unsweetened almond milk, my new swap for skim milk powder.

Date	Body weight (kg/ibs)	Daily calorie budget (kcal)	Breakfast	Lunch	Dinner	Snacks & drinks	Planned Exercise	Steps count-ed	Calorie balance / deficit (kcal)	Notes
08-Oct	74.2kg 163.6lbs	1047	Fat-free Greek yoghurt topped with dried cranberries, granola and honey (219kcal)	Chicken and kidney bean salad (217kcal)	Rice & beans with vegetable stew and air fried chicken (642kcal)		7 mins skipping (98kcal)	388	67	Yay! I'm back on the exercise train (hopefully).
10-Oct	74.2kg 163.6lbs	1047	Fat-free Greek yoghurt topped with dried cranberries, granola and honey (178kcal)	Chicken & coleslaw sandwich with chips (392kcal)	7 rice & grain with lentil, grilled hake & turkey (517kcal)	Crackers (50kcal)	7 mins skipping (98kcal)	183	8	"Can't be bothered." Tonight all I want is something to fill my tummy. I really couldn't care less if it's delicious or not.

Date	Body weight (kg/lbs)	Daily calorie budget (kcal)	Breakfast	Lunch	Dinner	Snacks & drinks	Planned Exercise	Steps counted	Calorie balance / deficit (kcal)	Notes
21-Oct	73.5kg 162lbs	1037	Toast (wholemeal medium white bread), coffee with skimmed milk(232kcal)	Pears, digestive biscuit (274kcal)	Freekah quinoa & spelt mixed pepper stir-fry with chicken (497kcal)			1175	34	Didn't get the chance to have a proper lunch today but I couldn't wait to try my hands on my new found mixed grain/swap for rice that I picked in store yesterday. it was worth it!
24-Oct	72.7kg 160.3lbs	1034	Fruit bowl (181kcal)	Wholemeal sardine sandwich (201 kcal)	Bulgur wheat, quinoa & wholegrain with vegetable stew, grilled hake & turkey (448kcal)	Low fat hot chocolate (39kcal)		3092	165	DRUM ROLL... I hit my target today! Created a new weight maintenance plan. This new plan with an increased calorie allowance will need some getting used to.

Looking back at this 30-day journal, the key call outs are:

1. You will occasionally drop the ball. There will be days when you are unable to weigh or log your meals and days you will forget to log your exercise or skip it altogether. Don't beat yourself up for it. Just get yourself back on track quickly and carry on.

2. Make a conscious effort to raise activity level in other areas e.g. take the steps instead of the lift on days you miss your planned exercise. You may have also noticed that I wasn't getting a full record of my daily steps because it's done through an app on my phone which is not on me all through the day. That's where a wearable tracker like a FitBit or smart watch would have come in handy.

3. Old habits die hard. I had a sweet tooth before I started counting calories and still do. That hasn't changed, the only changes are my choices (swaps) and portion sizes.

4. You may not get off to a good start like me exceeding my target on day one, losing half of my daily calorie budget to a poor selection of food and calorie-dense snacks. Your weight loss journey is also a learning journey. Start and learn as you go. If you are waiting until you know it all, you will never get started.

5. Never expect the magic to happen overnight. Your weight reduction will be gradual, some days it will stay flat, other days it may creep up again slightly. When it creeps up, honestly assess why and make adjustments. It is worth mentioning that body weight can also fluctuate each day due to water loss, e.g. your weight can fluctuate 1kg *(2.2lbs)* in one day, and it's not due to fat loss. You should try to weigh yourself at the same time each day to get a comparable measurement.

6. You are not restricted to a specific type of cuisine. I used to think weight loss was impossible with the Nigerian cuisine and could only be achieved with exotic food ingredients or Mediterranean cuisines. That's a myth. You can lose weight on any cuisine. Create the right balance of nutrients, adjust portion sizes and get creative.

7. You are not banned from relaxation and treats for life. Enjoy holidays, vacations and festive seasons but have a recovery plan and stick to it.

8. Remember, the amount of calories in a meal depends on both the amount of food and the calorie content of that food. The amount of food is very important and should not be overlooked. Make sure you enter the weight of the meal carefully in your app (or diet log). Small changes in

the total weight of your meals can have a large effect on weight loss success.

9. When you find meals and routines that work well, repeat them. Remember, we are creatures of habit and you can use this to your advantage. If you can successfully change your routines to include calorie control principles, you will find it much easier to stick to your plan.

10. Be disciplined. Whilst this is on your terms and in your own time, you will never get it done if you constantly make the habit of missing daily targets, skipping exercise, or not logging your meals. Limit the number of times you drop the ball.

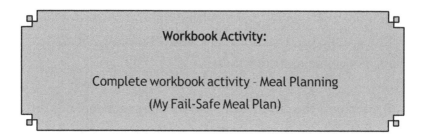

Workbook Activity:

Complete workbook activity - Meal Planning
(My Fail-Safe Meal Plan)

Measure It to Manage It

Well done for getting this far in the journey, even if only just reading for now to implement later on. This is the final but by no means least important aspect of your weight loss journey – tracking your progress.

As is said in management, you cannot manage what you do not measure. Documenting your meals and logging your weight daily is crucial to the success of your weight loss ambition. While eating well may seem the most crucial, the only way to know you are doing so is by measuring to assess the impact on your body weight and the other parameters.

Even when you think you have mastered the art of planning and cooking healthy low calorie meals, you still need to log these regularly to understand how you are progressing, establish what works for you and what doesn't.

If you are using an app, it will probably already be giving you graphs similar to mine below showing the speed of your progress and whether or not you are on track to meet your target by your set date. This gives you an early indication of your performance against target and the need to adjust or not.

Relying on your physical appearance only as a measure of progress can be deceitful and discouraging especially in the early days when the changes aren't yet visible. If your charts or records show things going in the right direction you can relax and stay focussed on your goal knowing the changes will start to be visible in a matter of time.

Another very good thing with tracking your progress if using an app is that it tells you what date you are likely to hit your goal based on your current performance.

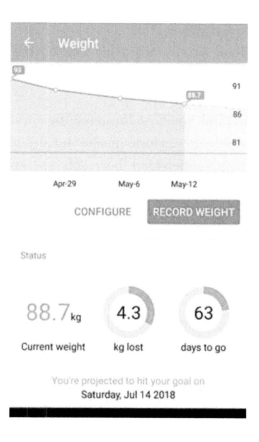

You should not look at your weight in isolation. It is also important to keep an eye on other weight-related goals (e.g. body fat, BMI), health goals (e.g. blood glucose, blood pressure), or body measurement goals (e.g. waist size, hip size) you may have set for yourself at the start. Whilst most of them will very likely follow the direction of your weight, it is not always automatic. I used to go into my local pharmacy weekly to use their more sophisticated scale to check my weight, body fat and BMI as well as regularly returning to the BMI calculator to see how my BMI was doing in relation to my goal of getting into the green zone.

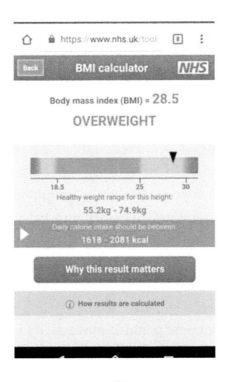

If your weight is trending in the right direction and the other goals aren't, then it is time to dive back into the records to see what patterns may be contributing:

- What are the foods I commonly eat on days I miss my daily target?
- What are the foods I commonly eat when I meet my daily target?
- Am I balancing my meals properly?
- Have I reduced calories but increased my intake of nutrients like cholesterol and sodium (salt)?
- Am I doing the right type of exercise to deliver on my body measurement goals?

These are some of the questions you may need to ask yourself and the answers should lead you to making the right adjustments. If there is a need to speak to your doctor for further guidance, then definitely do so.

Another reason I advocate the use of an app is that it gives you all of these useful insights based on what you have been logging.

Below is an example of what mine looked like at the time of writing. A few weeks ago, my weight as well as fat, saturated fat and cholesterol were pointing upwards, so I had to make adjustments again to my meals as it appeared I was dropping the ball and had been binging on snacks since I started working from home. My adjustments seemed to be working. My weight had gone down proportionately with the reduction in my fat and carbohydrate consumption but I was getting the least reduction in sodium. Knowing that high sodium levels increase the risk of high blood pressure, I looked further into the data to see what food was driving my sodium intake.

From my data below, soy sauce seems to be the main driver so I would need to either reduce the amount I'm using or swap for reduced salt soy sauce, for example.

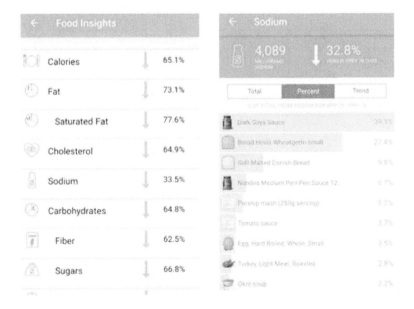

Irrespective of how you are logging your food and weight, whether manually or with an app, you will only be able to get quality insights if you have put in quality data. It is therefore highly imperative that you record, record and record. Quality data produces quality insights and helps you make quality decisions about your plan going forward.

Workbook Templates

Body Weight Tracker (Kilograms, Pounds & Stones)
Body Measurement Tracker (centimetres and inches)

THE WEIGHT LOSS CODE

Now You've Lost Weight, What Next?

CHAPTER 9

A NEW
NORMAL

There will come a time when you need to come out of active weight loss mode and work on holding onto your gains. I mean when your focus changes from losing weight to maintaining your new, healthy weight. As you can imagine, that also needs some degree of know-how. Even if you aren't there yet, it doesn't do any harm to know in advance and possibly have something new to look forward to.

I remember being told by a few people categorically that they were sure I would return to what I used to look like. Sarcastic statements like, "the smoothies and tablets will run out and we shall see." To date it still amazes me how many people thought it was their place to tell me what to do with my body, especially how many people were expecting the failure of that bold and positive attempt to lose weight. You will experience some of that. Even after you have reached your goal, you still need to stick to your guns, better still your 3Ds - Decision, Determination and Discipline.

So now you have achieved your weight loss goal, what next?

Calorie control does not stop when you achieve your goal; although how you approach it will change slightly. That is why I said at the beginning that this is not some diet fad, it is a lifestyle. Your relationship with food has changed and this is your new normal. It is now time to find your new WHY – why would you want to maintain this healthy weight?

Finding your new WHY requires you to look back and take an inventory of what you have learnt and gained on this journey. Those things will keep you going. For me:

- I stopped snoring from around the time I lost my first 10kg (22lbs/1st 8lbs) and never want to return to that.
- I am told I have cut ten years off my appearance. The truth is, I can see that in the mirror and I love the reaction when people hear my age. What woman doesn't love to look younger than her age?
- I am never ever going back to suffering thigh chafing and those burning lesions that come with it.

- I am not going back to those three muffin tops on either side of my tummy. If you don't know what muffin tops are, they are those folds on the side of the belly that look like skin bags.
- I am not going back to low energy levels and panting after walking up a few flights of stairs.
- I am not going back to those size 16+ clothes, especially now I fit perfectly in a 12 looking towards 10.
- Most importantly, I am never going back to red on the BMI scale, not even to amber. I am sticking to the green zone. There are so many health risk factors I don't have control over, but I do have control over my weight. Now that I have taken back that control, I am not prepared to lose it.

What are your new WHYs?

If you can see enough reason to carry on this lifestyle then you are on the right track to maintaining your new body weight.

Set a new goal:

Your goal now is different from what it was a few months ago and so will be your new daily calorie target. You now need to set a new goal using the same approach I taught you earlier in the book, with an important difference. This time, your current weight and target weight will be set as the same value.

Everywhere you chose to lose a certain amount of weight per week; you would choose to maintain your weight or a similar option depending on your app. If you are not using an app, you can also do this with the BMI calculator and the other methods I shared with you.

This should then give you your new daily calorie target. You'll be happy to hear it will clearly be higher and give you room to eat more. Don't go wild and crazy with that! The thought behind it is that you are now at a healthy weight and need to continue eating a healthy balanced diet within the recommended daily calorie intake and your personalised calorie target.

Keep planning, tracking and measuring:

Nothing good comes easy but by now portion control and meal planning should be second nature. It is advisable that you keep weighing and logging your meals if you want to. I still do when I can. However, if you have followed all the principles in this book and have reached this stage, your relationship with food will have changed positively and you are able to make the right food choices instinctively. You will most likely do more mental tracking but I strongly recommend that you maintain the habit of regularly checking your weight.

Things get even better:

You are now at a stage where you don't have to weigh ingredients and meals religiously anymore. The truth is, by now you have weighed so many meals and have a good idea of your ideal serving sizes without weighing. For instance, I know one serving spoon gives me around 150g (5.3oz) of cooked rice now without even weighing. You will find that you can accurately estimate portion sizes now, but ensure you continue to keep a close eye on portion sizes whatever way you choose to do it. I have stuck to weighing as much as is possible because it only costs me the time it takes to put my plate on the scale. You don't have to, if you have figured out the correct measures for your portion sizes using everyday utensils. You also need to keep monitoring your body weight and the other weight-related goals you set for yourself.

Know when to switch plans:

You need to be ready to occasionally switch back to weight loss mode when you drop the ball. Note I said when and not if. That's because even after you have achieved your weight loss goal, you still aren't perfect and situations where you cannot count, weigh, log or exercise will occasionally present themselves. The key is to plan ahead. For instance, on days I need to go for a meal out, I tend to have a smaller meal or skip a meal altogether prior to or after the outing to make allowance for the extra calories I might consume during the outing. I also do this on days when I need to taste many products at work as part of a taste panel. This is sometimes impossible especially during festive seasons and holidays. Those are the times you need to be quicker to react. If you notice weight gain, change your plan from a maintenance plan to a weight loss plan. Follow your new plan, switch back temporarily to weighing and logging meals until you get yourself back on track. Once you regain control, get on with your life

Keep exercising:

If there is good news and bad, when asked which I want to hear first I tend to go for the good news. The good news here is you can relax on weighing and journaling every meal. The bad news is you cannot stop exercising. At this stage the expectation is that you will appreciate the contribution of regular exercise to your achievement enough to make it part of your daily routine going forward. Regular exercise and physical activity are critical to holding your gains from this weight loss journey and will keep you in shape. Dropping the ball on exercising is giving an increase in body weight a free entry ticket.

Keep learning and swapping as you go:

Believe me, there is still a lot to learn even after you have achieved your weight loss goal. You will continue to discover new food items and more exciting swaps. It is a continuous learning process. As you may have noticed in my meal journal, I only discovered unsweetened almond milk towards the end of my six-month plan. I have discovered and will continue to find more even now. Last summer I stumbled on mango sorbet (73kcal per serving) in the frozen foods section of my local store and I was so excited to have found myself an occasional guilt-free treat. Guess what? This year I found a new range of low-calorie ice cream (68kcal per serving). Not in a million years did I think I would see that! In fact, it was something I used to joke about. You just need to stay curious. The food industry continues to be innovative and there are new products, trends and ideas landing on our shelves every day.

Above all, don't forget that we are creatures of habit. Enjoy good food but continue to take note of what works for you and repeat it. Not only was losing weight on your terms, keeping it off will also be on your terms. If you want to hold on to your newly-found body for the long term, you need to continue to do the right things, make the right choices, eat the right food, balance your nutrients and keep exercising. Not for another month, another six months, or another year but for life.

This is the new you and your new normal!

Your Next Step

Well done for coming this far. You have not only developed your own comprehensive, personalised weight loss plan without a personal trainer, but you have also started to implement your plan, and hopefully started to see the results.

I'd love to see you continue your weight loss journey, achieve your goal, and keep the weight off for life. So, stick to your plan and keep tracking and measuring.

You can continue to do this with your weight loss app. However, if you choose to track your progress manually, I recommend that you use the 'Weight Loss Code Breaker – 90 Days Calorie Control Journal'.

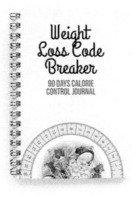

Get your journal now on *Amazon!*

OR

www.weightlosscode.co.uk.

My Journey
in Photo

I have shared so many tips in this book to help you on your weight loss journey but it is only fair to show you how these tips worked for me.

Writing a book was the last thing on my mind when I embarked on my weight loass journey, so these are my raw, real and unedited 'before', 'in transit' and 'after' photos.

Feel free to share your progress photos with me on my social media pages.

I am sure **YOU CAN DO IT!**

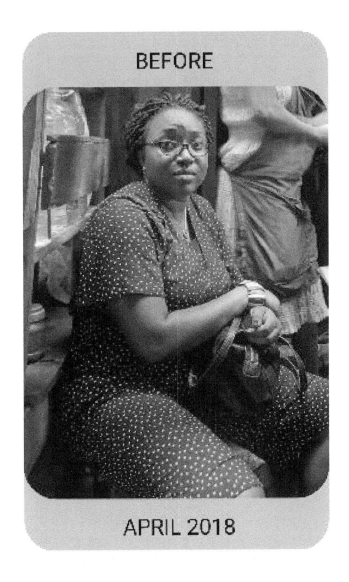

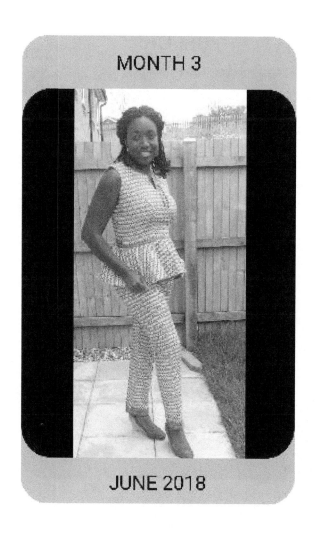

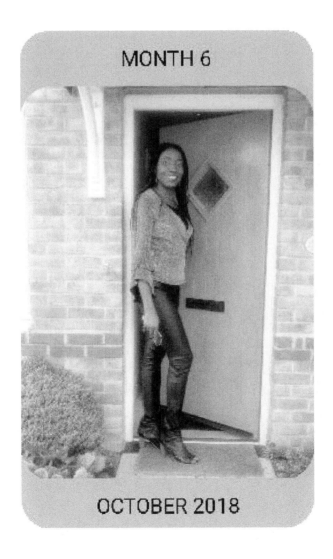

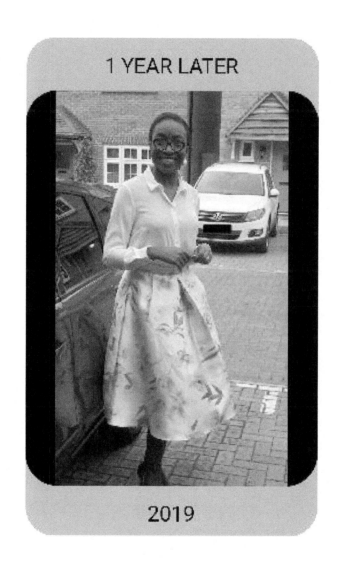

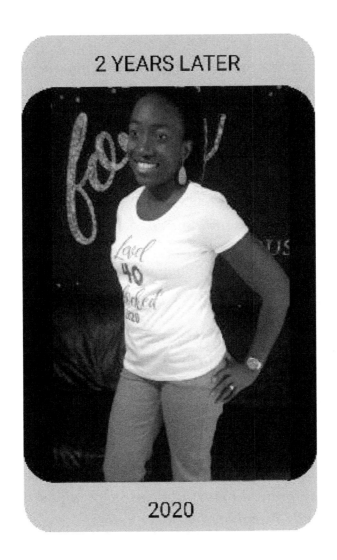

Useful Resources

- Public Health England: *https://www.gov.uk/government/organisations/public-health-england*

- British Nutrition Foundation: *https://www.nutrition.org.uk/*

- World Health Organization nutrition section: *https://www.who.int/nutrition/en/*

- Eatwell guide: *https://www.nhs.uk/live-well/eatwell/the-eatwell-guide/*

- NHS BMI Calculator: *https://www.nhs.uk/live-well/healthy-weight/bmi-calculator/*

- NHS Calorie Checker: *https://www.nhs.uk/live-well/healthy-weight/calorie-checker/*

- McCance & Widdowson Foods Dataset: *https://www.gov.uk/government/publications/composition-of-foods-integrated-dataset-cofid*

- American Journal of Clinical Nutrition: ***https://academic.oup.com/ajcn***

- Food calorie counter: ***https://caloriecontrol.org/healthy-weight-tool-kit/food-calorie-calculator/***

Reviews Make A Writer's World Go Round

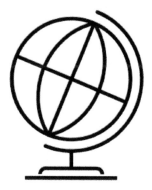

Thank you for reading my book!

I really appreciate all your feedback, and I love hearing
what you have to say.
I need your input to make the next version of this book
and my future books better.
Kindly leave me a helpful review on Amazon or any of
the other marketplaces where you purchased my book
and let me know what you thought of it.
Thank you so much!

-Yemi Fadipe

Printed in Great Britain
by Amazon